A Self-Fulfilling Prophecy: B
Successful Career in Health Research

A Self-Fulfilling Prophecy: Building a Successful Career in Health Research

SIMON STEWART

BA, BN, Grad Dip Ad Ed, PhD, NFESC, FAHA, FCSANZ

BICENTENNIAL

1807

WILEY

2007

BICENTENNIAL

John Wiley & Sons, Ltd

Other Wiley Editorial Offices

John Wiley & Sons Inc., 111 River Street, Hoboken, NJ 07030, USA

Jossey-Bass, 989 Market Street, San Francisco, CA 94103-1741, USA

Wiley-VCH Verlag GmbH, Boschstr. 12, D-69469 Weinheim, Germany

John Wiley & Sons Australia Ltd, 42 McDougall Street, Milton, Queensland 4064, Australia

John Wiley & Sons (Asia) Pte Ltd, 2 Clementi Loop #02-01, Jin Xing Distripark, Singapore
129809

John Wiley & Sons Canada Ltd, 6045 Freemont Blvd, Mississauga, ONT, L5R 4J3

Wiley also publishes its books in a variety of electronic formats. Some content that appears in
print may not be available in electronic books.

Anniversary Logo Design: Richard J. Pacifico

Library of Congress Cataloging-in-Publication Data

Stewart, Simon, 1964–
    A self-fulfilling prophecy: building a successful career in health research / Simon Stewart.
        p. ; cm.
    Includes bibliographical references and index.
    ISBN-13: 978-0-470-06071-1 (pbk. : alk. paper)
    ISBN-10: 0-470-06071-9 (pbk. : alk. paper)
    1. Medicine – Research – Vocational guidance.   2. Health – Research – Vocational guidance.
I. Title. [DNLM: 1. Health Services Research – methods.   2. Research Personnel.
    W 84.3 S851s 2007]
    R850.S76   2007
    610.71′1 – dc22

                                                                                          2006036939

A catalogue record for this book is available from the British Library
ISBN 13: 978-0-470-06071-1

Typeset by SNP Best-set Typesetter Ltd., Hong Kong
Printed and bound in Great Britain by TJ International Ltd, Padstow, Cornwall

This book is printed on acid-free paper responsibly manufactured from sustainable forestry in
which at least two trees are planted for each one used for paper production.

Table of Contents

Author Profile

Professor Simon Stewart is the Head of Preventative Cardiology at the world-renowned Baker Heart Research Institute in Melbourne, Australia. Integral to his role is leading a multidisciplinary team of researchers who are undertaking translational research and community-based trials in order to tackle the problem of cardiovascular disease across the whole 'life-time' spectrum of the disease. His research team and portfolio includes a number of newly appointed post-doctoral research fellows and plans for an indigenous research concentration working with local communities in the 'red centre' of Australia.

Through his extensive research collaborations both within Australia and overseas, Professor Stewart has been awarded honorary professorial appointments in health and medical research departments within Monash University (Preventative Medicine and Epidemiology), University of Queensland (Medicine), University of South Australia (Health Sciences), University of Adelaide (Health Sciences) and Deakin University (Nursing) in Australia, as well as the Chinese University of Hong Kong (Nursing) and University of Witwatersrand (Cardiology) in South Africa. He is an Inaugural Nurse Fellow of the European Society of Cardiology and an Inaugural International Fellow of the American Heart Association, and was the first-ever nurse to be awarded Fellowship of Cardiac Society of Australia and New Zealand.

Professor Stewart is world-renowned for his pioneering research and subsequent application of dedicated heart failure management programmes, publishing a series of studies involving more than 1000 patients and being published in *The Lancet* (1999), *Archives of Internal Medicine* (1998 and 1999), *Circulation* (2002 and 2006) and *European Journal of Heart Failure* (2005). In addition to co-leading international meta-analyses of heart failure management programmes published in the *Journal of the American College of Cardiology* (2004) and the *British Medical Journal* (2006), he has also been instrumental in applying these innovative models of care in Europe, the USA, Asia, South Africa and throughout Australia on a practical basis with a particular focus on creating sustainable models of funding for these programmes.

The National Health & Medical Research Council (NH&MRC) and National Heart Foundation (NHF) of Australia have continuously funded Professor Stewart's research via competitive grants and scholarships since 1995, including the prestigious Ralph Reader Overseas Post-Doctoral Fellowship Award, an Inaugural NH&MRC Clinical Career Development Award.

He has been awarded more than $AU7million in competitive research funding in the past five years on projects ranging from the Australian Research Council-funded Nurses E-Cohort Study of the nursing workforce in three different countries, to the National Health and Medical Research Council of Australia-funded Take Heart Study, examining ways to optimise the management of depression in patients being treated for chronic heart disease in the primary care setting. Professor Stewart is also co-Principal Investigator of what will become Africa's largest study of heart disease in a population in 'epidemiological transition' to more affluent disease states – the Heart of Soweto Study – and still actively collaborates with Professor John McMurray's world-renowned cardiovascular epidemiologic research group in Glasgow, Scotland.

As an active mentor, Professor Stewart currently supervises 10 full-time PhD candidates enrolled in a range of Australian universities. Seven of these candidates are supported by nationally competitive research scholarships and the remainder with competitive institutional scholarships. As part of the Heart of Soweto Study, Professor Stewart also co-supervises a number of PhD candidates from a range of African countries, working on various aspects of this project in Johannesburg, South Africa.

As part of his commitment to high-quality scientific publications, Professor Stewart was a founding Co-Editor of the *European Journal of Cardiovascular Nursing*, Associate Editor of the *International Journal of Cardiology* and is a peer reviewer for many prestigious journals, including *The Lancet, Circulation, British Medical Journal, Journal of the American College of Cardiology* and *European Heart Journal*. Since completing his PhD in 1999, Professor Stewart has published eight internationally distributed books. Over the same period, he has regularly published editorial, review and research articles in high-impact peer-reviewed journals. In the past five years, he has published more than 100 peer-reviewed articles and has a number of international research awards, including the American Heart Association's Martha Hill New Investigator Award (2000), for his pioneering research on nurse-led, multidisciplinary, heart failure management programmes.

Head, Preventative Cardiology,
Baker Heart Research Institute,
75 Commercial Road, Melbourne, Victoria 3004, Australia
PO Box 6492, St Kilda Road Central,
Victoria 8008, Australia
Telephone: +61 43 8302 111
Facsimile: +61 3 9521 1837
E-mail: simon.stewart@baker.edu.au

Foreword

Health and health services research is assuming increasing importance worldwide, but only a relatively few individuals build a successful career in the field. For those who wish to embark on such a journey, the road is often unpredictable, hazardous and painful. Many people who show early promise never fulfil their ambitions or achieve their true potential. This may be due to a variety of reasons, including personal ones, such as a lack of confidence, vision, energy or role model, or system or organisational ones, such as a lack of time, training, funding or other resources. The world of health research can be harsh and ruthless, with only the fittest surviving: it is full of individuals with strong personalities and ambitions and intense rivalries. Many people simply fail to survive because of poor planning, insufficient training, not having a mentor or support network or simply not working in a culture in which research is not only valued but is flourishing.

This book, therefore, is a welcome resource for the novice who aspires to become a successful health researcher. Written by someone with extensive experience and an international reputation in the field, it emphasises the importance of planning, strategy, mentorship and critical self-evaluation, and addresses neglected issues, such as completing doctoral and post-doctoral studies, benchmarking performance, publishing, presenting and interviewing. It is very much a practical guide and the author, in his usual frank and witty style, offers sound advice and useful tips which can enable the reader to succeed. Passion, enthusiasm, humour and good sense shine throughout. This book will be an invaluable resource to anyone intent on carving out a successful career in health research.

Professor David R. Thompson, BSc, MA, PhD, MBA, RN, FRCN, FESC, Director,
The Nethersole School of Nursing,
The Chinese University of Hong Kong,
Hong Kong.
davidthompson@cuhk.edu.hk

Preface

As is often the case, I was never really aware of how lucky I'd been in the early days of my research career and all the invaluable support I'd received to attain my career goals until very recently. As such, it was only when I was asked to share my experiences in developing a 'successful' research career by the School of Nursing at Deakin University that I was able to identify all the critical processes and pivotal events that conspired for or against my aspirations to make research a full-time occupation. For example, I was definitely not the number one choice for my first-ever job in research with my subsequent PhD supervisor and long-term friend and mentor Professor John Horowitz from the University of Adelaide in South Australia. Nor would I have landed in Scotland to undertake a post-doctoral research fellowship with another pivotal friend and mentor in my career, Professor John McMurray, if I hadn't been led to a short-cut to the train station on the last day of European Society of Cardiology meeting in Stockholm in 1997. These are past events that I had no control over. However, I am now able to reflect on the choices that I made that did have an enormous influence on my research career. In both of the instances mentioned above, I was challenged to step into the unknown and to make the most of opportunities that, at the time, made me extremely nervous. True to the maxim that the most interesting people are those that are prepared to take risks and continue to learn new things throughout their life, I've come to realise that these nerve-wracking decisions were pivotal to my career development. As such, they enabled me to put forward a diverse and competitive curriculum vitae relative to my immediate peers. I've also come to realise that I made a number of strategic decisions that, when taken as a whole, provided a strong framework for me to succeed not only in the short term, but hopefully in the longer term: only time and my peers will be able to judge whether I truly 'justified my existence' in the research world.

As someone who has been fortunate enough to be mentored by world-renowned cardiologists during my PhD and post-doctoral fellowship and, in more recent years, receive the invaluable advice and friendship of Professor David Thompson from the Chinese University of Hong Kong and Professor David Wilkinson from the University of Queensland (in their own right, world leaders in nursing and medicine, respectively), I have attempted to provide the same kind of support to emerging researchers who seek my help – not always with the same success but still with the same good intentions!

It is within this context that this book articulates all that I have learned about becoming a strategic researcher who has been able to *overachieve* by working smarter and more strategically than my otherwise more talented peers. It attempts to break down the key to a successful career in health research through a systematic analysis of what you can do to both improve your curriculum vitae and positively influence external factors that will determine the eventual success or failure of your career. As indicated by the title of this book, a successful career in health research is almost always a self-fulfilling prophecy. I make no apologies for relying heavily on my own experiences and efforts; nor am I ashamed for calling upon my network of PhD candidates and Post-Doctoral Fellows to provide their own insights on how they have developed their own research career (see Chapter 8). I merely present them as concrete evidence (warts and all) that it is possible to achieve something substantive if you are able to think and judge your career in a critical manner. I invite the reader to be as critical of the contents of this book as they would of their own endeavours.

Regardless of your opinion of this book, I wish you good fortune in carving out your own successful career in health research and making a significant contribution to your chosen area of interest and expertise by considering the advice I have offered and adapting it to your own vision for the future.

1 Becoming a Strategic Researcher: Increasing your Chances of Long-Term Success

INTRODUCTION

As its title would suggest, this book has been specifically written for the qualified healthcare professional (both junior and senior) who wishes to consolidate or build a successful career as a health researcher. However, as my research portfolio and responsibilities have expanded, so has my appreciation of those individuals (predominantly science and public health graduates) who have dedicated their careers to health research without undertaking specific clinical training. Not surprisingly, I have found that many of the career conundrums and issues that I have faced are the same ones that my fellow health researchers, irrespective of the presence or absence of a clinical background, have grappled with. This book's content and purpose, therefore, are not far removed from those individuals pursuing a purely scientific research career within the broad domain of health research.

It is within this context that this book outlines a range of strategies that will increase the probability of building a successful career in health research. Significantly, this book contains two key messages listed below that, despite their simplicity, are too often ignored by the average health professional considering an academic or clinical career with a strong research focus. This is not so surprising given the general lack of research culture and recognition of research within many emerging healthcare disciplines. It is a brave individual who declares their intention to adopt a different path from the majority of their colleagues and focus on becoming an expert in clinical research rather than a singular clinician – even if (as will be explored in Chapter 2) there needs to be a synergistic relationship between the two to achieve more effective clinical practice and better health outcomes. Given the inherent prejudices and ill-informed advice that such a declaration often attracts, a potentially promising career can easily lose momentum without careful consideration of what is required to achieve that career goal and how it can be reached with the minimum of external resistance and personal pain and suffering. Alternatively, there are those within historically strong health professions who are immune to the 'layers' of support and positive affirmation associated with their profession and somehow contrive to 'miss the boat' towards research success. It is for this reason that, regardless of your profession or area of expertise, you should carefully consider the following advice:

1. Plan your research career as early as possible – even if it involves initially focussing on developing ancillary skills and expertise (e.g. a nurse clinician with five years' full-time experience who then decides to take an interest in research).
2. Recognise the strategic importance of every facet of your professional activity in moving you towards achieving your ultimate goal.

It is important to recognise, at this point, that in most competitive circumstances (i.e. when you are competing with your peers for a position or funding support), selection panels will closely examine your curriculum vitae for clear links in the chain that are indicative of a progressive professional development into someone 'exceptional to the norm'. Not knowing, or indeed understanding, your personal history or circumstances, a selection panel will usually assume that you and your competitors have been given the same opportunities and attributes to succeed. What they will be searching for is that rare individual who demonstrates a single-minded purpose and determination to succeed: an individual who has not only worked on their strengths but conquered their weaknesses. If your curriculum vitae has 'winner' written all over it based on past accomplishments, it will foretell more success. Conversely, if it indicates past failures, you will have to work harder (if given the opportunity) to convince a panel verbally that there were either extenuating circumstances (e.g. you were raising a family or overcoming illness) or that you've changed your errant ways. Why, for example, should they select you to undertake a post-doctoral fellowship in a timely and successful manner and build towards a substantive research career when your PhD thesis was completed in a less than timely manner and/or had little or no impact – other than gathering dust on a library shelf?

Rather than wait until the completion of a higher research degree to reflect on your career direction, therefore, it is much better to plan at least two to three years ahead for the next crucial step and, in some cases, make long-term 'investments' that may not pay dividends in terms of your research career until five to ten years later. In this respect, there are a number of positive things and factors you can build into your personal plan to succeed as a researcher.

MENTORS AND ROLE MODELS

There are very few successful people who would not, at a moment's notice, be able to nominate the people who inspired, supported and/or cajoled them to excel. One of the most positive forces in my own career progression has been a select group of senior mentors who have fulfilled such a role to perfection at key points in time. Like all relationships, finding and maintaining a mentor to support you and your career is a two-way process that requires commitment from parties, involving a common purpose and direction in addition to mutual respect. As potent as such a relationship can be, it is important to note that 'pseudo or false mentors' (i.e. those who are prepared to use the relationship and your success to improve their own career!) are common and can prove to be a highly destructive force in your career.

It is vitally important, therefore, to recognise the common characteristics of a *positive* and true mentor who will support you for the right reasons:

- usually in a senior role similar to the one you wish to ultimately attain;
- preferably an international expert with good collaborative networks;
- achieved the type of things you want to achieve;
- comfortable in their own role, with nothing to prove in terms of individual success;
- readily acknowledge and demonstrate the role of teamwork;
- a good communicator;
- have or had their own mentors;
- not scared to support someone they consider to be more talented than themselves;
- prepared to accept that, one day, they might be asking you for a job!

Given the above list, in a positive mentoring relationship, your mentor will be prepared to:

- support you unfailingly in public;
- criticise and provide constructive advice in private;
- sacrifice their own needs for yours;
- recommend your services to peers;
- assist in any activities that further your career progression;
- persevere with you and affirm your career goals;
- tolerate irrational moments when all seems to be lost!

Of course, there is no 'dating service' for potential mentors and acolytes. However, as mentoring is considered to be a core component of being a successful academic or clinician, the best mentors are always searching for individuals who have good career potential and are prepared to spend the time making connections (even if they prove that there is no future in that particular relationship). Building a solid curriculum vitae in the early stages of your career and demonstrating the qualities of a 'winner' (as outlined) will undoubtedly increase your chances of being noticed and invited to discuss your career options with a promising mentor. In many instances, a mentor will also act as a PhD supervisor, but the two shouldn't be confused, as they can be mutually exclusive. Relying on one key mentor to assist you in your career development is fraught with danger given the inherent risk of illness, relocation or, indeed, a falling-out based on personal differences. In many cases, you'll find that a mentoring relationship will naturally evolve without either party's verbalising the underlying process that's taking place. However, given the risk of relying upon a single mentor, it makes sense to seek out a wider circle of mentors who can provide additional support.

Over time, a mentoring relationship will naturally evolve and mature much like any other relationship, particularly if you are able to close and, potentially, bridge the gap in career progression and achievements. The true test of a 'mentor–acolyte' relationship is, therefore, time and your ability to maintain a sense of respect and even reverence for the person who has helped you develop into the person/researcher you have become. Certainly, I have struggled at times to maintain 'equilibrium' with my earliest mentors. As such, the natural tension between developing an individual research identity and confidence has often clashed with a natural deference to a mentor's advice and opinions. However, like any good relationship, open and honest communication and empathy with each other's views and perspectives will always prevail, particularly if you are able to develop your own mentoring skills.

If many of the concepts and principles described above are similar to those found in 'self-help' books on building a healthy marriage or family relationship, it should come as no surprise. A positive mentor is worth the time and investment to weather changes in the circumstances and status of both parties. A false mentor, of course, should be quickly 'divorced', particularly if they exhibit any kind of abusive behaviour (e.g. taking full credit for your research, demoting you on the author list of an important paper or developing the next iteration of your research without providing you with the opportunity to progress your career).

A key component of a mentoring relationship is, of course, personal compatibility, common interests and, in many cases, a true friendship. Not every successful individual is, therefore, a potential mentor. In this context, learning from individuals who may possess a personality that clashes with your own but deserve your respect due to their ability to excel is also vitally important. Such 'role models' are usually much easier to find than a mentor with whom you are able to establish a true connection. The importance of such role models should not be under-estimated. If there is someone you are particularly impressed with and would like to emulate, try and find out how and why they have achieved what you admire. This may be difficult without 'cross-examining' them in detail, but by closely scrutinising what and how they do, you should be able to pick up important clues to improve your own success. For example, in my early clinical career as a cardiac nurse on a busy Coronary Care Unit, I was immediately struck by the calm and reassuring nature of the nurse in charge of the Unit. This was never more evident than when the inevitable 'cardiac arrest' of a patient occurred. While the attending nurses, cardiologists and anaesthetists alike typically created a heady cocktail of stress and urgency that could easily suck the unwary (including yours truly) into a sense of panic and disordered thinking, this particular nurse (who always exuded a sense of calm and authority) would immediately take control and ensure the best of emergency care was delivered. Although I never had the chance to talk through how and why he was able to become the 'calm eye of the storm' in the Coronary Care Unit (he was a very taciturn and private person), I certainly aspired to exude the same sense of calm and mastery when confronted with emergency situations. It was only a few years later, after I had spent many hours learning my advanced life support skills and successfully coordinated the resuscitation of two patients who had simultaneously suffered a cardiac arrest (one patient undoubtedly scared the other to 'death' by suddenly collapsing and turning blue) with only one resuscitation cart and, therefore, one set of equipment, that I felt that I had mastered some of what this earlier 'role model' had shown me through actions much more powerful than the spoken word. I immediately remembered to calm and focus my thoughts and actions many years later (i.e. long after leaving a clinical role), when I was the first to arrive on the scene of a 'head-on' vehicle accident with multiple casualties and more recently when coping with two seriously ill passengers on a long-haul flight without immediate medical support.

Remaining calm and focussed in the often hectic process of beating a deadline for delivering a research application on time is an attribute/goal I've consistently aspired to as a result of my 'emergency' experiences and, of course, one of my earliest role models – the 'icy calm' charge nurse of the Coronary Care Unit. It is in this way that role models, even when they touch your life only briefly, can have a profound and lasting impact on you, your career and your overall view of the world. Role models obviously require less investment in time and energy, but may well yield similar positive results in building a successful research career.

POSITIVE PEER RELATIONSHIPS

No one will really understand what you are experiencing and striving to achieve more than your peers in the research world. The term 'research world' is probably most appropriate in this context given that you are most likely to derive the greatest benefits from establishing and maintaining contact with researchers on a national and international basis as opposed to local level, particularly if there is a scarcity of researchers from your own discipline. Despite some differences, the process of undertaking a higher research degree and striving to move on to a productive post-doctoral position that will lead to a permanent research position is the same the world over. Rather than treating every individual in your immediate area of expertise as a rival or enemy to be despised and destroyed in case they outperform you and successfully compete for funding or a key position, it is more productive to form strategic partnerships that will assist you to achieve your short- and long-term goals. This may sound dramatic, but the research world is littered with individuals who strive to dominate rather than collaborate. Many overly competitive researchers spend precious time and energy working out ways to unravel a colleague's career rather than spending it constructively on their own endeavours. To succeed, focus on improving yourself, not denigrating your peers! If you are on the end of someone's vitriol or machinations, take it as a compliment and remember to stay focussed on what you can control and achieve. Forming relationships with international peers (usually at international conferences) is particularly useful and has the potential to facilitate the following:

- being introduced to their own mentor(s), who may well be international experts in your field of research and may facilitate an academic visit in the future or peer-review your next research article;
- undertaking an academic visit at another research institution;
- developing a collaborative research project;
- jointly publishing review papers;
- keeping up to date with the latest research developments or opportunities for research funding;
- sharing strategies and ideas to further develop your research skills and output;
- providing moral support at key moments (e.g. presenting at a large scientific meeting);
- arranging an overseas post-doctoral fellowship.

In the longer term, there is a strong possibility that at least one of your peers will become an international expert. Future collaborations with such a person, particularly with a track record of papers and projects over a long period of time, will provide you with greater access to research funds and/or the potential to generate a larger number of publications in high-impact journals.

HOT RESEARCH TOPICS

As will be discussed in greater detail in later chapters, without a long-term career plan, many promising researchers consign themselves to failure from the beginning by choosing, or allow themselves to adopt, a mundane or routine research programme that is never going to be published in high-impact journals (see Chapter 8) or attract invitations to speak at international conferences. Quite naturally, many novice researchers regard the opportunity to undertake a PhD as the defining moment of their research career and that everything will take care of itself thereafter. However, long after the glow of self-satisfaction in achieving the hard-earned reward of being called 'Doctor' has dimmed, many researchers are left to ponder why their 'passport' to research success has been rejected at the next border. In the majority of cases, this will reflect the fact that a novice researcher has been 'lost' within a large research programme and their research is either 'owned' by their principal supervisor or is unlikely to make any immediate impact synonymous with the candidate themselves.

As indicated above, a long-term strategic plan that looks beyond a PhD and focuses on post-doctoral studies is the best antidote to an 'impulsive' decision to accept second-best offers to undertake a research programme that will ultimately support the career of an established researcher or larger research programme – in essence, avoiding a 'PhD factory' run by 'false or pseudo mentors' who are still striving to specifically further their own research career.

ACTIVE PROFESSIONAL ENGAGEMENT

Standing out from your peers naturally takes time and commitment. It not only involves working harder and smarter on your research, connecting and collaborating with your research peers (regardless of their health or scientific discipline), but also becoming professionally active in a range of ways that might include:

- becoming a formal and active member of a relevant professional organisation;
- volunteering for committee duties;
- organising local to international scientific and educational meetings;
- registering as a journal peer reviewer in your area of expertise;
- regularly attending scientific meetings and asking critical questions during symposia;
- assisting in the compilation of expert guidelines.

Despite the time and commitment required, all of the above represent good long-term investments to access specific research funds for pilot research projects, travel funds to attend larger scientific conferences, invitations to join editorial boards of national and international journals and, ultimately, to professional recognition as invited Fellowship to a prestigious professional organisation.

As always, it is important to avoid working for one specific organisation and, therefore, choosing a careful balance of discipline-specific organisations, larger non-discipline-specific organisations that provide access to a range of health professionals and prestigious international organisations that may take longer to engage with. Clearly, working for professional organisations will facilitate your ability to meet and collaborate with your peers and meet potential mentors and role models.

RAPID CAREER PROGRESS

One of the major quandaries in building a research career is 'part-time versus full-time PhD/higher degrees'. A straw poll of ultimately successful researchers, regardless of the discipline, will provide you with a strong hint – always choose the fast track to attaining your goals! Unfortunately, in many health disciplines, the former has proven to be more popular. There are many reasons why part-time PhDs have proven to be more popular:

- The underlying research culture of many clinically based disciplines favours individuals who appear to retain their 'clinical credibility' whilst undertaking research: they can't be accused of turning their back on their profession.
- Psychologically, part-time is less of a 'commitment' to a research career – it leaves greater room to withdraw with dignity in case of failure.
- Full-time funding is often difficult to obtain.
- The demands of family and a social life appear to be best met by part-time status.

The last, in particular, is a major fallacy, given that a part-time PhD equates to up to eight years of juggling the two 'masters' of work and study compared with three years of concentrating on a single goal, often, with careful planning, providing a flexible workload that is more amenable to family life. It is important to stress, once again, that successful researchers often take the harder, less travelled road to success. This means completing a succinct and productive PhD and then maintaining a highly productive career path. If we individually address the four issues raised above, it becomes clear how completing a full-time research apprenticeship is nearly always preferable to becoming successful in the longer term:

1. *Create your own research culture!* Remember that selection panels/quality mentors are always looking for something different. If you are younger and have developed your research career more rapidly, you'll be ahead of your competitors from the very beginning.
2. *He/She who dares wins!* If you are suffering from a crisis of confidence when entering a PhD, you clearly haven't the personal attributes and mentoring support to complete the long and arduous journey.
3. *Quality research attracts funding!* If you have planned your research career properly, you will already be competitive for internal or external scholar-

ships (most of which have tax advantages and allow you to work on a casual clinical basis to provide a solid income) and with appropriate mentoring, good supervisors and cutting-edge research, should ensure you are in a position to undertake your PhD full-time.

4. *Short-term pain equals long-term gain!* As already noted above, faced with three compared with six to eight years of hard work and life disruption as part of a PhD candidature, most sane people would opt for the former. Apart from the fact that six to eight years will magnify the usual feelings of hopelessness and lack of progress associated with a PhD, it will place you a good three to four years behind your competitors who adopt a full-time approach.

As will be expanded upon later, even when undertaking a PhD full time, many candidates mistake volume for quality and, perhaps more importantly, the ultimate purpose of the PhD itself. In this context, it is vitally important to remember that a PhD thesis (particularly if it takes the form of a traditional volume of more that 200 pages) is not the defining product of your efforts: people don't weigh a thesis to determine how good you are and everyone ends up with same honorific and three-letter initials. In actual fact, it is the personal and research qualities you have developed during the process that determine the overall quality of your PhD.

What does this mean in practical terms? First, if you can learn and acquire the qualities of an independent researcher within a couple of years and can produce a thesis that passes scrutiny, plan to submit as early as possible rather than writing pages that will lie dormant on your shelf for years to come! In this respect, it is preferable to produce a thesis via published research reports that both force you to be succinct and to the point and provide external validation via external review: it would be a brave examiner indeed who rejected concrete evidence that you've made the grade by publishing your research in a quality, peer-reviewed journal! Once you've established a pattern and reputation of rapid progress, it will become a self-fulfilling prophecy for you to be labelled as someone on the 'fast track' and given further opportunities to rapidly progress in your research career.

SUMMARY

There are many factors that can work either for or against you in trying to develop a successful research career. You need to be aware of the factors that are represented in Figure 1.1 and develop a framework of positive factors to support your career. In the same context, it is important not to become overwhelmed by unavoidable negative factors or become too concerned with your 'competitors' (other than benchmarking your progress and/or building

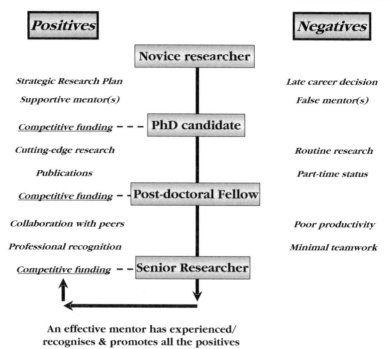

Figure 1.1. Positive and negative factors that impact on an emerging research career

constructive relationships – see Chapter 4). By creating a favourable environment for success by selecting the right people to support you (e.g. mentors and peers), the right research (e.g. internationally competitive), expanding your sphere of influence through high-profile professional activities and, finally, taking the fast track to productivity, you are more likely to succeed. Ultimately, success is almost always a self-fulfilled prophecy.

> **Key Points: Plan your research career as early as possible – even if it involves initially focussing on developing ancillary skills and expertise. Recognise the strategic importance of every facet of your professional activity in moving you towards achieving your ultimate vision for your career.**

2 Critical Self-Analysis and Personal Improvement: Do I Currently Have the Skills and Knowledge to Become an Expert Health Researcher?

INTRODUCTION

In an increasingly competitive world, it would appear that the soul searching and torturous preparations typically associated with selecting and securing a prosperous and rewarding career are becoming the exclusive domains of school children – the premise being that the earlier the preparation, the greater the likelihood you'll have the grades to select which university degree or training programme you'd like to undertake and the world is your oyster from that point onwards. Paradoxically, of course, the days of entering a single profession and focussing on a single role for a lifetime of rewarding employment has long been replaced by calls for a 'flexible workforce' and 'multi-skilling', with an emphasis on discovering how to learn and readily access information in preparation for a range of jobs, rather than focus on specific skills and knowledge. Certainly, modern funding models for universities and independent research institutions in many developed countries, with their increasing emphasis on revenue raising via entrepreneurial activities and less emphasis on providing 'core' funds, provide less security for their employees than ever before. This is often compounded by an increasing focus on individual, performance-based contracts that allow the institution to dictate who and what is valuable to them in a much shorter timescale (e.g. over three- to five-year terms). On a more positive note, this new reality means that there are actually more career options for relatively young adults than ever before, particularly for those prepared to take the challenge of life-long learning and development. Moreover, whilst there is certainly an undercurrent of ageism once someone reaches their forties (i.e. barring them from adopting a completely new career challenge), this 'invisible barrier' is likely to dissolve in the ageing workforces of developed countries and provide new career challenges for individuals prepared to accept them.

How does this 'brave new world' impact on someone wishing to pursue a career in health research – does it hinder or help? Overall, it most probably helps, for two concrete reasons: first, because it reinforces the idea of 'multi-skilling' and preparedness to take on new roles (i.e. it creates an environment and stimulus for potentially talented researchers who are already expert clinicians or clinical educators to take on a new career direction) and, secondly, because the 'window of opportunity' to take on a new career direction is widening to include individuals in their thirties, forties and even fifties.

On a more specific level, in the medical (e.g. clinical medicine and basic medical research) and the healthcare disciplines (e.g. nursing, physiotherapy, pharmacy and occupational therapy), there is an increasing 'blurring of the lines', as the traditional and rigid roles of the past are replaced by more prag-matic ones that deal with our ever-increasing ability to prolong life and its common by-product, chronic disease, in more flexible ways. There is also an inherent value placed upon the combination of clinical experiences, advanced training and tertiary qualifications in enabling someone the ability to claim 'expert' status. Naturally, the evolving nature and diversity of contemporary medicine and healthcare, in addition to the active support of individuals con-tinuously acquiring new skills and knowledge, provide a rich environment for motivated individuals to build rewarding and innovative careers based on the single goal of improving the lives of others, whether it be at the individual or societal level.

One of the most important and challenging roles in an evolving disease and healthcare environment is that of the career researcher. This book obviously deals with the strategies that will increase your chances of building a successful care in healthcare/service research. However, as indicated above, any profes-sional career in health requires a dedication to life-long learning and develop-ment. Figure 2.1 also shows that a health career is not simply about clinical practitioners and their clinical practice in promoting health and effectively treating disease, but the body of knowledge and skills that underpin their practice via high-quality research and the effective communication of health-care messages to the public and new knowledge and skills to healthcare pro-

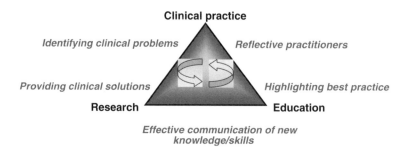

Figure 2.1. The critical nexus between clinical practice, education and research

fessionals. Simply focussing on only one aspect of this important triad of clinical practice, research and education will effectively disable one's ability to harness the synergy between these three critical activities and therefore make a substantive impact on health outcomes. More importantly, it demonstrates that the pathway to an effective career in health research can be found via all three activities. This is the most natural and common pathway derived from an initial career as a trained healthcare professional with a number of years of clinical experience and, knowingly or not, active involvement and exposure to research and educational activities.

As noted in the introduction, it is largely on this premise (i.e. the qualified healthcare professional who wishes to consolidate or build a career as a health researcher) that this book outlines the strategies that will increase the probability of success in the field of research. This particular perspective assumes, therefore, that you have most probably already built up a formidable knowledge base plus a range of experiences and skills that will enable you to tackle a research career with confidence. The first step in building a successful career in research is to *critically reflect* on your strengths and weaknesses and how you can use them as a strong foundation to ultimately succeed in clinical research. For those individuals who are approaching this from a different perspective (e.g. from a more scientific and less clinically focused background), the same imperative to evaluate your strengths and weaknesses apply, particularly if you wish to engage in more clinically based research.

CRITICALLY EVALUATING YOUR STRENGTHS AND WEAKNESSES

Consistent with Figure 2.1, showing the critical nexus between clinical practice, education and research, it should come as no surprise that the most successful clinical researchers typically possess the following three qualities:

1. clinical expertise (and therefore credibility and insight) relevant to their specific health discipline;
2. broad range of research skills/expertise that enables them to select and apply appropriate research methods to answer a broad range of clinical issues/problems;
3. good communication/education skills to convey their ideas and findings and inspire others to follow their lead.

Whether you agree with this list or not, or indeed the strategies outlined throughout this book, there is little doubt that a dispassionate and highly critical appraisal of your strengths and shortcomings as a clinician, educator and researcher will increase in intensity as you attempt to improve your status from novel researcher/trainee to more senior roles (i.e. post-doctoral fellow, independent investigator and dedicated research professor). Any perceived weaknesses will be magnified and highlighted when competing against your peers for an ever-dwindling number of places at the top of the academic pyramid. Before embarking on the rigorous process of career advancement, it makes perfect sense to reinforce the positives by using the following strategies, where appropriate:

- translating expert clinical or educational practice into formal clinical and tertiary qualifications (e.g. Graduate Certificates/Diplomas or Masters Degree);
- making the effort to engage with professional organisations (both national and international) to obtain official Member or Fellowship status;
- demonstrating a willingness to incorporate research into your role as an expert clinician by becoming actively involved in formulating/reviewing clinical guidelines and/or facilitating clinical research activities;
- formalising other areas of interest and skills that are outside of your immediate discipline (e.g. undertaking formal qualifications in business management or education) that still have relevance to becoming an effective critical thinker and productive worker.

On the other hand, it also makes perfect sense that you address your initial weaknesses in order to improve the value of clinical research training and to compete for competitive research funding to effectively kick-start your career and mark yourself as a winner from the very beginning. This may be achieved by following the strategies below, where appropriate:

- participating in small-scale research studies, with the prospect of becoming increasingly involved and being included as a named author and/or investigator in funded research;
- assuming a specific research role (e.g. coordinator/data-manager) within large-scale clinical research studies, with the prospect of developing ethics applications, receiving advanced training in good clinical practice and being audited to ensure that the quality of research is high and any results are valid;
- undertaking initial research training programmes (e.g. Graduate Certificate in Public Health).

As outlined in Table 2.1, there are many miscellaneous skills/attributes that can be acquired and will pay handsome dividends during a long-term research career. For example, if one considers the art and science of presenting an important research paper at a major international conference, there are distinct advantages in being able to engage and inspire a large expert audience, effectively convey your key messages with your words, slides and graphical representations (see Figure 2.2 as an example) and answer a range of questions, both specific to your research and its overall implications at the health service/population interface, with confidence. Being multi-skilled in this regard will provide you with the same confidence to face an intensive selection panel

Table 2.1. An array of attributes of that will improve your effectiveness as a researcher

Attribute	Purpose
Effective public speaking and presentations	You may have the best research in the world, but if you cannot communicate its importance and potential impact in public, it will likely be ignored. Alternatively, less talented researchers with better public persona will dominate your field, overshadow your work and become successful. Remember, people respond to passion! There are many courses that can help you dissect your own style of presentation, and cover the basics such as lighting, sound and the basic principles of effective slide presentations. One of the most confronting aspects for most people is public speaking and, perhaps worst of all, being taped or filmed. If you want to be successful, you will need to conquer such fears early and make a positive out of a potential negative.
Debating skills	One of the most impressive speakers I've ever been privileged to hear present on the international stage is Professor David Celemajer from the Heart Research Institute in Sydney, Australia. It comes as no surprise that he is a debating champion, given his ability to tackle the prevailing viewpoint and provide a more than cogent interpretation that challenges the audience to think again and re-evaluate their own interpretation of the current state of play. Scientific debates, whether a formal part of a programme or part of the usual question time during an abstract session or scientific symposium (which can be extremely confronting in front of a 'gladiatorial' audience who sense a weakness and support the one or two 'bullies' who typically love asking tough questions), are an integral part of a researcher's world. Once again, a potential strength can be turned into a positive. Even if you are confronted by an 'intellectually' superior opponent, you can often win a debate by presenting your ideas in a simpler, more appealing and more gracious manner.
Creative and scientific writing skills	Consistent with the above, the written word plays an integral role in conveying the importance of your research. At the most critical level, a well crafted and worded research paper is more likely to be given a second chance if there are scientific issues to be addressed, while a difficult-to-read paper will be rapidly rejected on the premise of sloppy presentation equals sloppy science. Although more difficult to convey via the written word, passion for a particular subject or piece of research is likely to invoke a positive response. This is a good reason to gain mastery at both ends of the writing spectrum: technical and creative.

Table 2.1. *Continued*

Attribute	Purpose
Advanced computing skills (e.g. word-processing and statistical packages)	As each new iteration of Microsoft's (and other ubiquitous software companies') latest operating system and programs appears, there is a natural tendency to cling to the old and simpler ways of interacting with our 'personal' computer; everyone knows that each new advancement to simplify tasks simply complicates them. However, it is essential, for work efficiency and research leadership, that you master key areas of computing. This includes advanced word-processing, statistical analysis and, increasingly, graphic and presentation packages.
Effective use of wider forms of information technology: beyond computers	Despite the information technology revolution, many researchers are still scared of new technology and are unable to utilise it to enhance their research and educational activities. The internet and mobile communications offer many opportunities to rapidly access new knowledge, disseminate findings and organise/coordinate diaries and workloads. Efficiency and innovation, when combined with natural talent, are unbeatable combinations!
Building and maintaining large databases	Beyond mastery of the many forms of data-processing programs driven by ever more powerful computers is learning to create and maintain large databases that: (a) capture the 'reality' of what is being researched at the coalface (e.g. within a hospital clinic), (b) accurately store study data in a readily interrogator-friendly form, and (c) provide the right form of data that can directly or indirectly (via transformation/modification) address your research questions or hypotheses and generate meaningful results.
Graphic design (see Figure 2.2)	'A picture tells a thousand words.' We hear this particular piece of wisdom in many contexts, but I wonder how seriously many health researchers listen to this simple message when sitting through scientific conferences! A good presentation with the appropriate mix of words, colour and graphs to translate often complex messages into simple ones is extremely powerful.
Fast touch-typing	One of the simplest, most effective techniques to improve your efficiency as a researcher is to increase the speed at which your thoughts are transferred to the computer screen. Touch-typing is a fundamental (but often unfashionable) skill that can have a profound effect on the speed and sophistication of your writing skills. The emerging alternative, of course, is voice-recognition systems that allow you to convert your speech into words on the computer screen. At a personal level, I have always preferred to use my inner 'narrative' voice to write and therefore prefer to type my thoughts directly onto the page. Irrespective of the vehicle, it makes sense to improve the transfer of your expertise and thoughts into the written form.

Table 2.1. *Continued*

Attribute	Purpose
Using advanced reference programs	One of my fondest memories of a very senior and world-renowned physiologist, who still worked in the cardiac laboratory as I undertook my PhD studies, was his manipulation of a card system to keep track of key references for his latest publication and his ability to refer to the exact results of relevant experiments in the literature. Of course, possessing an enormous intellect and memory is a rare talent. For the rest of us 'mere mortals', it is imperative to use a system that keeps track of the literature we have read and facilitates the creation of a current and incisive list of references: as a reviewer, I am immediately unimpressed by an introduction that misses key papers in the literature and assume that such 'sloppy' referencing extends to the study someone is describing!
Advanced statistical analyses	Dove-tailed with the ability to manage large datasets (never an easy task) is the ability to undertake advanced statistical analyses. This does not in any way devalue the role of dedicated biostatisticians and, indeed, the more advanced functions provided by modern statistical packages. It simply provides you with advanced 'discriminatory' powers to design your research appropriately, deliver statistically relevant data and accept or reject the advice of statisticians (notoriously unable to agree amongst themselves!) and the often misleading results produced when a statistically naïve individual plays with a powerful statistical tool.
Understanding public health/ epidemiological principles	Ultimately, most, if not all, research (even if it is the most basic of research, exploring the cellular mechanisms underpinning a particular pathological process) will be evaluated on the basis of its immediate or future impact on the overall health of whole populations. This is why research applications inevitably ask what health issue it is linked to and how it will ultimately benefit society (particularly within current research priorities). Unfortunately, such a simple and fundamental question often proves to be a grant application's weakest link. At a more advanced level, many projects rely upon recruiting large numbers of patients or subjects. Clearly, mastery of public health and epidemiological principles will improve a critical aspect of many research proposals.
Health economics	A major focus of healthcare systems and budgets under increasing financial pressure from more expensive therapeutic options is health economics. Being able to integrate a sensible and understandable health economic component in clinical health research is a major advantage. As always, it would be a mistake not to collaborate with a highly regarded health economist (I'm

Table 2.1. *Continued*

Attribute	Purpose
	more than fortunate to work with Professor Paul Scuffham from Griffiths University in Australia, who was trained at the 'home' of health economics – the York University) but your interactions are likely to be much more fruitful if you are able to interact in a meaningful way and understand key principles underlying economic analyses.
Good communication skills at the individual level	It seems obvious that research is mostly a 'team' game that requires good communication and motivational skills in order to improve productivity and creative synergy. Not everyone is a natural-born communicator. Fortunately, there are personal-development courses that can enhance your ability to connect and work productively with other people.
Conflict resolution	Unfortunately, good communication and leadership skills do not automatically protect you from conflict. Conflict over the direction of a study, intellectual property or something as simple as order of authorship on a research paper is inevitable in teams of researchers who are all trying to achieve and progress their careers. Acquiring good conflict-resolution skills may prove to be particularly useful in navigating large research concentrations in which 'conflict' and competition are viewed as the norm.
Multidisciplinary teamwork	Confining oneself to a single discipline in today's research environment is tantamount to career suicide in most instances. Opening a dialogue with experts integral or even peripheral to your area of expertise in order to better understand their 'view' of a particular health issue is critical to multidisciplinary research. As a precursor to collaboration, there are always texts and short courses aimed at the novice level that will enable you to better understand and appreciate another health or related non-health (e.g. education) discipline.
Critical-thinking strategies	When immersed in a particular project, research concentration or problem, it is often hard to escape a certain mentality or perspective. This has certain advantages if it enables you to communicate in the same way and contribute to a single focus. Yet, being able think outside of the square and critically examine all facets of your activities in a critical and constructive manner are extremely useful skills, not only in terms of developing new and innovative research directions, but also presenting 'balanced' reports. As with 'sloppy' introductions, I'm always amazed how even senior researchers can produce an otherwise stimulating and provocative research paper without paying close attention to detailing their studies' obvious limitations. Once again, there are many courses that develop

Table 2.1. *Continued*

Attribute	Purpose
	critical-thinking strategies that enable an individual to 'attack' a problem from many different angles; including from the inside out and from a wholly external perspective.
Developing leadership skills	There are very few natural-born leaders and, indeed, a large majority of individuals who would prefer not to assume responsibility for other people. Unfortunately, it is often difficult to develop a successful research career without assuming some form of leadership, so why ignore this 'weakness' if you are uncomfortable with the thought of assuming responsibility? Career progression is often judged on your increasing ability to assume responsibility for increasingly larger and more complex activities (i.e. from coordinating a small study in a hospital clinic to a multi-institutional programme). Leadership doesn't have to involve assuming a formal title, but does involve providing direction and stimulating people to agree and cooperate. Once again, there are many courses that can develop your ability to 'lead' others in an effective manner.
Business management	As indicated earlier in this chapter, there is an increasing focus on entrepreneurial research activities that generate wealth as well as new knowledge. Accompanying this trend is the increasing realisation that managing any form of research activity requires careful planning, risk assessments and projections on future gains and outputs. Most research organisations now use strategic and business plans to guide their activities in a sustainable manner. Naturally, all of these concepts are closely aligned with running a business and mastering business management is an extremely useful way of distinguishing oneself from the 'ordinary' researcher. Two of the most successful and respected researchers I've had the pleasure to work with (Professor David Thompson from the Chinese University of Hong Kong and Professor Andrew Coates from the University of Sydney) possess MBAs and have consistently demonstrated their ability to apply their acquired skills and knowledge both directly and indirectly to their research activities.

when attempting to sell your credentials and visions for funding or for a specific research position. Many of the attributes listed in this table do not require formal training and/or can be developed through self-directed learning activities and dedicated short courses. This, of course, is the beauty of a commitment to life-long learning and taking advantage of better understanding the process of acquiring new skills and knowledge as an adult.

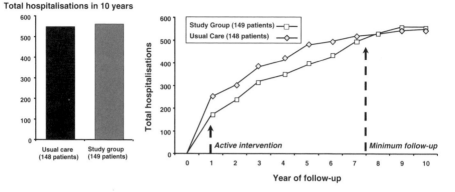

Figure 2.2. Compare and contrast: the importance of maximising the immediate and lasting impact of your pictures/graphs

Legend: Consider the two panels based on the same data from a recent research report on the impact of a multidisciplinary, home-based intervention on hospital readmissions on two groups of patients over a 10-year period. The left-hand panel presents these data in bar-graph form and would require some explanation of what happened over time to produce a similar result and to pique the audience's interest. Alternatively, the right-hand panel clearly tells a story that requires little explanation.

SUMMARY

Before embarking on a research career and preparing your first application for competitive funding, it makes sense to give yourself an immediate advantage relative to your peers by presenting the best possible curriculum vitae. This usually means being exposed to quality researchers and research projects that will immediately provide you with an idea of what it will take to succeed and, hopefully, give you a sense of the immense satisfaction that a researcher gains from entering an international fraternity that gather in different (and usually beautiful) parts of the world and also contribute to better health outcomes for your community. It also makes sense to critically reflect on your strengths and weaknesses and continually work on the latter (usually throughout your career) to turn them into your strengths. As indicated by Table 2.1, there are a myriad of attributes (not necessarily confined to those immediately associated with research and your specific discipline) that contribute to a successful research career.

Consider that one single inspirational presentation given to an audience that has an invited international expert may open the door to gaining an invitation to speak at an international conference that they are organising, or a visit to their institution, or the opportunity to write a chapter in the latest book that they are editing. Consider also the possibility of speaking to someone in a tea room about your mutual research interests and recognising the possibility of collaborating and making the sum of your research efforts greater than your independent efforts. Finally, consider discovering a future research 'star' who will trust and collaborate with you for many years to come just because you were able to solve a simple statistical or technological problem for them early in their career. All of these scenarios are based on real-life examples and illustrate the potential to maximise your interactions with people, machines and whole institutions to make the most of your research career. As with most careers, it is not usually the individuals with the greatest intellect who succeed, but those who are the most strategic and make the most of their talents.

Key Points: There are close links between the triad of clinical practice, education and research in designing and applying successful healthcare treatments and strategies. Successful researchers recognise the need to become experts in all three areas and develop a broad range of skills and domains of knowledge to assist them to become more effective in all aspects of their diverse role. Successful researchers turn their weaknesses into strengths.

3 Benchmarking your Capabilities and Performance: Improving your Chances of Success within a Competitive Environment

INTRODUCTION

Once you have looked inwardly and critically appraised your own strengths and weaknesses and determined what it will take to reinforce and address them, respectively, it is time to look outwards and examine the research environment you hope to conquer. It would be reasonable to suggest that most researchers are passionate about their research and its potential impact. Rather than money and fame, their passion for making a difference is a major stimulus for choosing and persisting in a research career (see Chapter 8). As discussed in the previous chapter, it is also reasonable to suggest that the most 'talented' or scientifically intelligent researchers are not necessarily the ones who have successfully navigated their way to the top and hold the most prestigious research positions. A key question, at this point, is whether it is possible to both succeed and stay true to the passion for the research that led to such a career. Fortunately, the answer is a resounding yes.

Apart from the most brilliant researchers who don't really have to try to succeed but are immediately recognised by their peers and mentors (and, therefore, earmarked for rapid career progression), what distinguishes one researcher from the next when all things are otherwise equal in terms of career progression and success? As indicated earlier in Chapter 1, it's all about *strategy, strategy and even more strategy*! The most successful researchers make the most of their intellect and ideas, work on both their strengths and weaknesses and then employ a strategic plan to ensure that they are competitive in all the key indices of a successful research career:

- personal scholarships/fellowships;
- competitive research funding;
- accepted and invited presentations at international conferences;
- peer-reviewed publications;
- professional awards/prizes.

The remainder of this book will focus on specific aspects of the above list and a range of strategies that can be employed to achieve success. However, in order to create and then apply a successful strategic plan, it is essential to generate realistic and useful targets that neither leave you short of success nor create an unsustainable and undesirable imbalance in your life that leaves little room for other important activities (e.g. your family and social activities) and/or destroys your original passion for your research. Fortunately, you are not the first, nor will you be the last, person to build a research career. The relative success and failures of your peers (particularly those who are at the same stage in their career or have followed the type of career path you wish to follow) represent a particularly important resource for you to both judge your current status and plan for the future. Regardless of whether you wish to follow a unique vision and forge your own path within your own discipline(s), it is highly desirable that you strategically assess your immediate and 'future' (i.e. those who have taken the next step – from PhD to Post-Doctoral Fellow) peers to compare your progress against to ensure that you are always aiming to exceed the 'benchmarks' that they have set.

BENCHMARKING YOUR CAREER PROGRESS

Intuitively, we are all aware that the term 'success' (defined by the Cambridge Dictionary (*http://dictionary.cambridge.org/*) as 1. '*the achieving of desired results*' or 2. '*something that achieves positive results*') can only be framed within the context of various forms of failure relative to a 'successful' outcome. However, there is ample anecdotal evidence to suggest that many health researchers are completely unaware of what it will take to succeed and, as a result, do not have a strategic plan to attain such success. As indicated above, in a competitive world (particularly one such as research that relies on peer reviews at nearly every stage to determine the relative merits of funding and publication), it is vitally important to know the levels of expertise and outcomes that you need to attain in order to be considered a success. As an added bonus, such success will often reap additional rewards, whether they be related to money, status or, probably most importantly, to the amount of recognition your research ultimately attracts and the overall impact it has on improved health outcomes.

In simple terms, it is strategically important for you to 'benchmark' yourself against your peers in order to determine whether you, relative to the same stage of research career, are:

- *Currently under-achieving*: this simply means that you do not have the same demonstrable attributes and skills as your immediate peers. At the novice stage, this would render you non-competitive for a PhD scholarship and would attract less interest and fewer offers for support and exciting research projects from potential supervisors/mentors relative to your competitors. Ideally, you would address such 'under-achievement' as rapidly as possible or simply hope that you are lucky enough to fall into a highly successful research group that will, through the team output and reputation, build your research career for you. Naturally, in such a team, you are likely to be the 'work horse' and be overlooked for career progression and rewards.

- *An average researcher*: as the term 'average' suggests, means that your profile and accomplishments are roughly equivalent to the vast majority of your immediate peers. As a PhD candidate, about to complete your formal programme of research, it would leave you in a neutral position as far as your future career progression and competitiveness to take the next step via a competitive post-doctoral fellowship are concerned. As above, you may be fortunate to establish a successful post-doctoral position by being swept up by a busy and successful research team that requires a coterie of workers to handle a large volume of research activity in a proficient manner.

- *A highly competitive researcher*: this means that you've outperformed the majority of your peers. At the post-doctoral stage of your research career, you would have already achieved a number of things (e.g. completed a highly successful PhD, published numerous articles in high-impact journals and attracted competitive funding) that would mark you as someone who is capable of taking on more senior research roles, worthy of competitive funding and, most importantly for your future career, an attractive proposition to promising novice researchers who are looking for successful mentors to guide their career. Whether you stay competitive is really up to you. I have met quite a number of 'high flyers' who have assumed that they would naturally progress and continue to perform. This may be through the combination of taking 'safe' options (e.g. not being prepared to move out of their comfort zone and work with a new team or learn new skills) or, in many cases, over-estimating their abilities and output relative to the knowledge and skills that they have acquired under a highly supportive mentor/supervisor: in other words, as soon as you take that person out of a successful environment and research stream that provided relatively easy opportunities to perform at the highest level (e.g. high-impact peer-reviewed research reports), they are unable to maintain even a fraction of the same output.

It is within this context that Figure 3.1 provides a practical example of the *relative* levels of research success in terms of the most common indices used by peer-review and promotion panels to rank and reward individuals at the initial stages of their research career. The significance of your career progress and achievements is most notable when actually competing against your peers for research support (see below). Importantly, therefore, it is important to remember that there is nothing stopping you from improving your

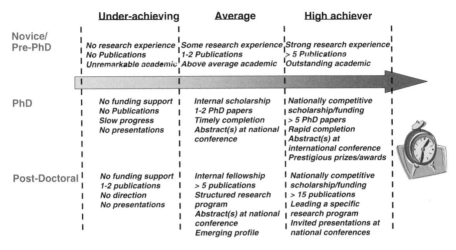

	Under-achieving	Average	High achiever
Novice/ Pre-PhD	*No research experience No Publications Unremarkable academic*	*Some research experience 1-2 Publications Above average academic*	*Strong research experience > 5 Publications Outstanding academic*
PhD	*No funding support No Publications Slow progress No presentations*	*Internal scholarship 1-2 PhD papers Timely completion Abstract(s) at national conference*	*Nationally competitive scholarship/funding > 5 PhD papers Rapid completion Abstract(s) at international conference Prestigious prizes/awards*
Post-Doctoral	*No funding support 1-2 publications No direction No presentations*	*Internal fellowship > 5 publications Structured research program Abstract(s) at national conference Emerging profile*	*Nationally competitive scholarship/funding > 15 publications Leading a specific research program Invited presentations at national conferences*

Figure 3.1. Benchmarking your progress to become a 'high achiever'

competitiveness (i.e. from a 'below average' prospect to a highly successful post-doctoral research fellow) at each stage of your research career: this book obviously outlines the strategies that can assist you to improve the quality and impact of your research. Clearly, it is much better to critically examine your progress at an early rather than later stage of your career. However, the imperative to do so can be stimulated by discovering and becoming passionate about a new research topic. As such, the phrase 'better late than never' is very relevant and most peer reviewers and panels recognise a 'passion' for what it is, rather than focussing on the age or stage of the individual.

IDENTIFYING YOUR CAREER TARGETS

Once you have made the decision to 'benchmark' yourself against both your immediate (at the same career stage as you) and future (i.e. preparing for the day when you have completed your PhD and are seeking post-doctoral funding) peers/competitors, there are many ways you can build a comprehensive picture of what it will take to succeed. This includes:

- talking to experts in your field of research, discussing their career progression, seeking their advice on what you need to achieve in the current research and funding environment and identifying other key individuals in the field who are worth contacting and/or researching (see below);
- searching the World Wide Web for the home pages of successful researchers relevant to your chosen area of endeavour: these pages often list publications, presentations and competitive research funding in addition to a chronological account of their career progression;

- running specific publication searches (e.g. Medline or PubMed) on key individuals to determine the pattern (i.e. number of publications per annum) and range of papers that they have produced;
- talking to and researching competitive funding bodies, both internal and external, to determine what criteria they use to rank applicants and identify specific individuals who have previously succeeded in gaining support for further research (see specific section below);
- attending national and, if possible, international conferences in order to gauge the quality of research and those presenting with a specific focus on 'new investigator' and prize sessions relative to your stage of career;
- reading relevant peer-review journals to determine the standard of research that is regularly published and attracts positive editorials;
- joining peer-support groups in order to compare experiences and advice relating to career progression;
- acting as peer reviewer for scientific journals or meetings.

Although this may appear to require a substantial time commitment, it is worth noting that if you are really interested in building a substantial research career, it is worth spending a few hours every couple of months or so to undertake vital research that will help you achieve your ultimate goal. It is also worth noting that benchmarking your competitors and thereby honing your curriculum vitae and overall competitiveness should become a routine activity throughout your career.

PROFILING YOUR COMPETITORS/PEERS

If you are truly intent on being competitive for prestigious milestones in your career progression, you will use the above strategies to closely examine those who are achieving what you want to achieve in the next step of your career (i.e. successfully competing for post-doctoral research funding) and then try to emulate or exceed what they have achieved at the same stage of their career.

As an example, Table 3.1 examines the broad profile and achievements of a cross-section of typical applicants[1] for prestigious post-doctoral fellowships relating to clinical and public health research in Australia and internationally, provided by the National Health and Medical Research Council of Australia for 2007 onwards, from the perspective of an independent peer reviewer. Any examination of their individual competitiveness has to be couched in terms of the specific intent of these awards and the criteria used by impartial peer reviewers to rank applicants, usually on an initial basis of competitive (worthy of support) versus non-competitive (unworthy of support, even if unlimited

---

[1] In order to protect the confidentiality of applications to this scheme, original details have been changed and a 'typical' profile of early career researchers compiled.

funding were available) and then ranked according to merit. Their competitiveness is also dependent on their chosen field of research relative to the
national health priorities established by the Australian Federal Government
in collaboration with the peak health bodies (including the Australian Research
Council and the National Health and Medical Research Council).

UNDERSTANDING THE BACKGROUND TO RESEARCH: AUSTRALIA'S NATIONAL PRIORITIES IN FUNDING HEALTH RESEARCH

As indicated above, any examination of the competitiveness of an application
to a national funding body has to take into consideration not only the specific
intent of the award (this is detailed below) but also the overall national context
of health research. In Australia, like many other countries, research is often
(but not exclusively) driven by strategic plans and priorities. In reviewing an
application for personal support, there is a natural tendency to initially judge
the importance of the individual's proposed research stream relative to national
health priorities; it obviously helps if they clearly identify with key issues and
closely link their research with 'national' benefits. As stipulated by the Federal
Government   (*http://www.dest.gov.au/sectors/research_sector/policies_issues_
reviews/key_issues/national_research_priorities/priority_goals/promoting_
and_maintaining_good_health.htm* (accessed September 2006)) in Australia,
there are four priority areas for funding and support (see text box).

Australian Health Research Priorities

1. A healthy start to life

*Counteracting the impact of genetic, social and environmental factors which
predispose infants and children to ill health and reduce their well being and
life potential.* Human health in the developing foetus and in early childhood
is critical to the future well being of the adult. Research shows that health
and well being in early childhood is predictive of later positive outcomes,
and that health in middle and late childhood is also crucial. This goal supports the Government's *National Agenda for Early Childhood* initiative.

2. Ageing well, ageing productively

*Developing better social, medical and population health strategies to improve
the mental and physical capacities of ageing people.* Australia's population
is ageing, with a significant projected increase in the number of people aged
over 65 and over 85. While Australia is relatively well placed compared
with many OECD nations, major shifts in cultural expectations and atti-
tudes about ageing are necessary to respond constructively, at both an
individual and population level. A healthy aged population will contribute

---

actively to the life of the nation through participation in the labour market or through voluntary work. This goal supports the Government's *National Strategy for an Ageing Australia.*

3. Preventive healthcare
New ethical, evidence-based strategies to promote health and prevent disease through the adoption of healthier lifestyles and diet, and the development of health-promoting products.

Preventive healthcare research will improve the prediction and prevention of disease and injury for all Australians through the adoption of healthier behaviours, lifestyles and environments. Research will generate an improvement in the design, delivery and uptake of programmes such as exercise-based rehabilitation. There are several major disease targets amenable to immediate study, such as cardiovascular health, neurodegenerative diseases, mental ill-health, obesity, diabetes, asthma and chronic inflammatory conditions. Research on prevention will emphasise interdisciplinary approaches, including research on ethics, drawing on contributions from the social sciences and humanities, as well as from the health and medical sciences. It will also focus on developing new health-promoting foods and nutraceuticals. This goal supports the Government's *Focus on Prevention* initiative.

4. Strengthening Australia's social and economic fabric
Understanding and strengthening key elements of Australia's social and economic fabric to help families and individuals live healthy, productive, and fulfilling lives. Living in today's society involves a complex web of choices, yet many of the traditional support structures are weaker than they have been in the past. Enabling people to make choices that lead to positive pathways to self-reliance and supportive family structures is more important than ever. The interactions between the social safety net, social and economic participation, financial incentives and community and private sources of support are critical in helping people maximise their potential and achieve good, healthy, lifetime outcomes. In the decade ahead, it will be vital to understand and support the drivers for workforce participation and the broader social and economic trends influencing Australian families and communities. This goal supports the Government's welfare reform and participation agendas. Research in this area will emphasise interdisciplinary approaches, drawing on contributions from the economic, behavioural and social sciences.

These priorities form an integral part of the background of health research and it would be foolish to ignore the major forces influencing health research in Australia or any other country (e.g. that dictated by the National Institutes of Health in the USA).

PURPOSE OF PERSONAL SUPPORT: THE NHMRC
POST-DOCTORAL TRAINING FELLOWSHIPS

Anyone applying for one of Australia's most prestigious Post-Doctoral Fellowships (whether they be a general Public Health Fellowship or a particularly named Fellowship such as the CJ Martin Fellowship), as in any other country, would be wise to carefully examine the underlying purpose and intent of their award and tailor their career (as part of pre-planning) and application accordingly. Those researchers profiled in Table 3.1, therefore, would have read the following when first contemplating applying for post-doctoral support on the organisation's website (*http://www.nhmrc.gov.au/index.htm* (accessed September 2006)):

> 'The purpose of NHMRC Training (Postdoctoral) Fellowships is to provide opportunities for Australian researchers to undertake research that is both of major importance in its field and of benefit to Australian health. Training (Post-doctoral) Fellowships provide a vehicle for training in basic research either in Australia or overseas (where appropriate), to enable Fellows to work on research projects with nominated advisers. Awards are offered to a limited number of persons of <u>outstanding ability</u> who wish to make research a significant component of their career.
>
> To be eligible to apply, applicants must hold a doctorate in a health related field of research or have submitted a thesis for such by 31 December of the year of application. Applicants should have demonstrated an interest in, and ability to pursue, a career in research and be currently engaged in such activities. At the time of application, applicants should not have more than two years' postdoctoral experience from the date that the doctoral thesis was passed.'

A major goal underlying many of the post-doctoral fellowships provided by this scheme (with a success rate as low as 20 per cent of all applicants) is the progression of an individual researcher from their *original* research group and research area to a new research group that provides an environment in which the newly qualified researcher will continue to learn and expand their research skills and contribution to their chosen field of research (although it should be noted that some researchers successfully argue for a complete change in research focus by clearly demonstrating their passion and potential for career growth). What it doesn't 'reward' is those who wish to stay in their comfort zone of research and continue a close relationship with their original research supervisor and mentors and/or exactly the same stream of research (unless the latter is a natural progression). Unfortunately, many researchers fail to read the purpose and intent of the funding scheme and fall at the first hurdle through a 'technical' disqualification or at the final hurdle when a peer-review panel is forced to choose between those who are truly forging a new path and training opportunity compared with those who are moving to a new team on paper only.

SCORING INDIVIDUAL APPLICATIONS

As with any other funding scheme, there are comprehensive guidelines for reviewing and scoring applicants for National Health and Medical Research Council of Australia Training Fellowships, that take account of the individual profile and potential of the applicant (40 per cent), the major research stream/ project that they will focus on (20 per cent) and the impact of their research from a professional, scientific and translational perspective (40 per cent). In this instance, the researchers profiled in Table 3.1 were judged via a written application and a series of referee reports from past and proposed supervisors/mentors as well as an independent report. In other schemes, it is usual for an applicant to 'pass' an initial inspection of a written examination and referee reports and then compete with other 'outstanding' candidates at an interview.

THE INDIVIDUAL Criteria: **Undergraduate/Honours/Other Degree** Research Experience Professional Skills Potential to succeed Prizes/Lectures/Conferences Organised/Courses	
Total	**40 POINTS**
PROPOSED RESEARCH & ENVIRONMENT Criteria Component 1: Quality of Project and Potential Benefits – (10 points) Criteria Component 2: Supervisor/Institution – (10 points)	
Total	**20 POINTS**
RESEARCH QUALITY & OUTPUT Criteria: Quality and Quantity Originality	
Total	**40 POINTS**
OVERALL SCORE OUT OF 100 POINTS	....

Table 3.1. Typical profile of early career health researchers in Australia and key points from the peer-review process

Gender	Age (years)	PhD	Broad area of research	Notable publications	No. of citations	Quality of group & institution	'X' factor score (passion & impact)	Notes
Female	35–40	7yrs	Biomedical research	13 research papers	–	Internationally renowned	8 out of 10	Good combination of research output in specialist journal and quality research and research group
Male	35–40	4yrs	Human movement	13 research papers	–	Specialist centre of research	5 out of 10	Combination of quality research and output with specific research group
Female	40–45	Pending	Mental health	8 research papers	39	Internationally renowned	9 out of 10	Very good combination of papers in journals with good impact factors, citations in specialist journals and quality research group
Male	35–40	1.5yrs	Medicine	12 research papers	23	Internationally renowned	6 out of 10	Publications in specialist journals with no outstanding output. Quality research group
Male	40–45	1yr	Infectious diseases	12 research papers	–	Internationally renowned	7 out of 10	Publications in specialist journals with low impact factors. Quality research group
Female	35–40	1.5yrs	Neurosciences	1 research paper	–	Internationally renowned	2 out of 10	Low research output (with some potential expressed). Quality research and group

Female	35–40	2yrs	Nutritional sciences	5 research papers	—	Nationally renowned	6 out of 10	Modest research output, but papers in good impact factor journals. National leaders in field of research
Female	25–30	<1yr	Human disability	3 research papers	—	Nationally renowned	4 out of 10	Low research output in specialist journals combined with national leaders in research field
Male	30–35	Pending	Cardiology	3 research papers	—	Nationally renowned	7 out of 10	Low research output to date combined with nationally renowned research group
Female	35–40	<1yr	Nutritional sciences	7 research papers	—	Nationally renowned	8 out of 10	Modest research output with nationally renowned research group
Male	40–45	1yr	Psychology	20 research papers	—	Nationally renowned	9 out of 10	Good research output in specialist journals. National leaders in field of research
Male	40–45	1.5yrs	Environment health	13 research papers	—	Nationally renowned	5 out of 10	Good research output in high-impact specialist journals. National leaders in field of research
Female	25–30	<1yr	Physiology	1 research paper	—	Nationally renowned	5 out of 10	Low research output. Modest research group
Female	50–55	1.5yrs	Paediatrics	7 research papers	15	Internationally renowned	8 out of 10	Modest research output given low-impact, specialist journals. Internationally renowned research group
Female	25–30	3yrs	Psychology	8 research papers	—	Nationally renowned	7 out of 10	Low research output given low-impact journals and reviews. Nationally renowned research group

Table 3.1. *Continued*

Gender	Age (years)	PhD	Broad area of research	Notable publications	No. of citations	Quality of group & institution	'X' factor score (passion & impact)	Notes
Female	35–40	<1yr	Cognitive–behavioural sciences	2 research papers	–	Nationally renowned	2 out of 10	Low research output. Modest research team
Female	25–30	<1yr	Psychology	29 research papers	–	Nationally renowned	9 out of 10	High-impact research in top specialist journals. National leaders in research area
Female	35–40	2yrs	Psychology	7 research papers	50	Internationally renowned	7 out of 10	High research output given one high-impact paper plus good impact factor journals. Internationally renowned research group
Male	50–55	2yrs	Public health	7 research papers	–	Nationally renowned	7 out of 10	Reasonably high research output given publication in top specialist journals. National leaders in research area
Female	20–25	<1yr	Physiology	6 research papers	–	Nationally renowned	8 out of 10	High research output given high-impact journals, although many 'team' publications. Nationally renowned research group
Female	35–40	2yrs	Genetics	12 research papers	149	Internationally renowned	10 out of 10	Excellent research output given high-impact papers and citations. International leaders in research area

Female	25–30	2yrs	Respiratory medicine	14 research papers	—	Nationally renowned	8 out of 10	Good research output in specialist journals. National leader in research area
Female	35–40	<1yr	Paediatrics	3 research papers	—	Internationally renowned	4 out of 10	Low research output. Internationally renowned group
Male	45–50	2yrs	Microbiology	40 research papers	70	Nationally renowned	9 out of 10	Very good output despite large number of review papers. Many papers in high-impact specialist journals. National leaders in research area
Female	45–50	Pending	Public health	3 research papers	—	Nationally renowned	5 out of 10	Modest research output in specialist journals. National leaders in research area
Female	35–40	<1yr	Endocrinology	8 research papers	—	Internationally renowned	8 out of 10	Excellent research output in very high-impact journals. World leaders in research area
Male	35–40	2yrs	Psychology	12 research papers	—	Nationally renowned	7 out of 10	Good research output: large number of papers pre-PhD research. Nationally renowned group
Female	35–40	<1yr	Epidemiology	16 research papers	—	Internationally renowned	9 out of 10	Very good research output in specialist journals. World leaders in research area
Female	40–45	1yr	Community health	13 research papers	—	Nationally renowned	6 out of 10	Modest research output given low-impact journals. Nationally renowned group

Table 3.1. *Continued*

Gender	Age (years)	PhD	Broad area of research	Notable publications	No. of citations	Quality of group & institution	'X' factor score (passion & impact)	Notes
Female	30–35	<1yr	Behavioural sciences	5 research papers	–	Internationally renowned	7 out of 10	Very good output given one very high-impact journal paper. Internationally renowned group
Male	25–30	Pending	Behavioural neurosciences	4 research papers	–	Internationally renowned	7 out of 10	Excellent research output given all papers in high-impact journals. World leaders in research area
Female	25–30	3yrs	Anatomy/physiology	3 research papers	–	Internationally renowned	1 out of 10	Modest research output in specialist journals with potential for improved output. Internationally renowned group
Female	35–40	<1yr	Gastro-enterology	7 research papers	–	Nationally renowned	6 out of 10	Good research output in specialist journals. National leaders in research area
Female	35–40	2.5yrs	Neurophysiology	13 research papers	–	Nationally renowned	8 out of 10	Very good research output top specialist journals. National leaders in research area
Female	40–45	<1yr	Human movement	2 research papers	–	Nationally renowned	3 out of 10	Low research output in low-impact journals. Nationally renowned group
Female	25–30	<1yr	Physiology	12 research papers	–	Nationally renowned	7 out of 10	Good research output in specialist journals. National leaders in research area

PICKING THE WINNERS

A close inspection of the typical profile of early career health researchers in Australia (Table 3.1) reveals a number of important points (at the very least in terms of competing for prestigious Post-Doctoral Fellowships in health research in Australia):

- Those attempting to consolidate/establish a competitive clinical research career are typically aged 30 years or more, having spent a considerable number of years establishing their credentials/qualifications in their specific discipline.
- Many applicants are in the process of reapplying for a Fellowship (having failed to obtain funding in the first instance following PhD completion).
- There is a healthy proportion of female Australian researchers competing for these awards, having juggled the dual responsibilities of career and parenthood.
- There is a healthy diversity in the depth and breadth of research being proposed. However, this makes it difficult to assess and makes reference to 'research priorities' and specific intentions of the grant very important.
- Those who have managed to publish more than 10 research papers (particularly in high-impact journals – either specialist or general) are more likely to be competitive. However, opportunity relative to age and employment (particularly for those new to the research environment) is an important caveat and one particularly high-impact paper can be extremely important.
- Many researchers are unaware of the importance of checking how many times their papers have been cited.
- Working with national and world leaders in the chosen field of research is extremely important to differentiate one's self from other researchers.
- The 'X-Factor' in terms of general impressions from a written application (and, in some cases, interview) should not be under-estimated. This really stems from the applicant's ability to 'capture' the interest of the peer reviewers and compel them to argue for funding support. This is usually based on the idea of career trajectory, the person's underlying passion for their subject and, of course, their potential to make a substantive difference.

Picking the winners (i.e. those individuals who are automatically placed in the top 5–10 per cent of their peers) is difficult without viewing the specific applications and referee's reports, but it is obvious that some applicants compel a review panel to support them because they are passionate about their career and research, have obvious career potential as leaders in their field of research, are researching a 'hot' topic, have already demonstrated high research output and impact, and propose to join world leaders in their field of research.

SUMMARY

A strategically aware researcher will know exactly what is required to become competitive at the local, national and international levels. They will tailor their research activities and training to ensure that they exceed the benchmarks established by their peers. This requires becoming actively involved in a range of activities in which you are able to monitor the progress of your 'current' and 'future' peers, building strategic alliances and always thinking carefully about the next step in your research programme. It is worth noting, once again, that benchmarking your curriculum vitae to better compete against your peers does not require you to actively work against them; unfortunately, the temptation to spend more time worrying about others and place obstacles in their way is all too common. Setting mutual goals and establishing supportive relationships that are likely to become more important as you reach more senior positions form a much more positive and strategically sensible plan than making enemies throughout your career.

Key Points: As indicated by the title of this book, regardless of your inherent talents and qualifications, there are many things you can do to create a successful research career if you are aware of whom and what you are competing against and what you have to achieve in order to place yourself in control of your own destiny. However, as indicated by the alarm clock in Figure 3.1, there is a narrow window of opportunity for you to prove yourself a 'high achiever' and worthy of funding and career support (usually within two to three years of completing a PhD).

---

4 Choosing the 'Cutting Edge' of Health Research

INTRODUCTION

It will be reiterated throughout this book that without long-term career plans, your chances of ultimately succeeding and attaining (or, indeed, exceeding) your original goals are greatly diminished. Importantly, this doesn't mean that your career has to be a carefully managed affair: having a strategic plan means that you have thought about what you want to achieve and that you are more likely to recognise a golden opportunity (even if it has its inherent risks) to build an *extra-ordinary* career. It is within this context that many promising researchers consign themselves to failure from the beginning by choosing, or allowing themselves to adopt, a mundane or routine research programme that is never going to be published in high-impact journals (see Chapter 8) or attract invitations to speak at international conferences. Without these indicators of your relative value on the national and international stage, your ability to convince a selection panel and your peers that you are worthy of more senior research positions and sustained funding for your research programme is reduced.

Unfortunately, given that your PhD and/or post-doctoral studies will often take years to reach fruition and advances in your chosen area of interest are almost inevitable, you almost need to be clairvoyant to guarantee that you are publishing and presenting novel findings that will make a suitably large and recognisable impact. Unless you are prepared to take your chances and simply hope that your chosen area of expertise will lead you to the top, it is imperative to carefully choose an initial area of research that will both make an immediate impact and provide you with a chain of investigation that will sustain your research career for a number of years.

IDENTIFYING A 'HOT' RESEARCH TOPIC

Before considering the specifics of choosing an area of research on which to base your career, it is extremely important to understand the 'big picture' issues that impact on the health of communities throughout the world; this has already been touched upon when reviewing Australia's pre-designated national health priorities in the previous chapter. As the clinical practice and knowledge domains of health disciplines span the whole continuum of conception to death and from health to illness, there is obviously an enormous array of health research topics to choose from. However, choosing a highly specific research topic that will lead to dramatic results in a small group of individuals has to be weighed against working on producing modest results in a large group of individuals, particularly if that research resonates with health priorities prospectively identified by governments, funding organisations and health providers. The trade-off, of course, is that becoming an international expert in a highly specific area of health research is likely to be easier when competing against a few individuals compared with competing against many individuals who are focused on more popular areas of research.

From a global perspective, as the overall wealth of the world's population steadily increases, there is an inevitable trade-off, with a parallel increase in the total burden and impact of more 'affluent' disease states. These disease states mark a transition in human history from the preponderance of traditional killers of malnourishment, infectious disease and violence that severely limited life-expectancy to 'self-inflicted' conditions that emerge in the latter years of an expanded lifespan. Such a phenomenon has been exacerbated by advancing treatment options that merely prolong the inevitable in an ageing body rather than provide an 'immortality elixir' that defies the natural ageing process once the inherent risks of being young are successfully navigated.

Figure 4.1 synthesises World Health Organisation data showing the most common causes of disability and premature mortality in both men and women around the world. Clearly, undertaking research that provides practical and cost-effective solutions (the economics of health are becoming increasingly important!) to address the multitude of problems that they engender at the individual and societal levels will obviously be viewed as important and treated as high-priority for financial investment (i.e. research grants and service development funds) and publication. In most developed countries, the progressive ageing of the population has meant that there has been an enormous interest and dedicated research funding directed towards the following:

- coordinated disease management programmes to deal with an increasing number of individuals with chronic disease;
- primary prevention strategies designed to minimise the number of individuals developing a chronic condition;
- community models of care designed to minimise the most costly component of healthcare expenditure (hospitalisation), e.g. hospital-at-home programmes for patients with malignant disease and non-institutional mental healthcare programmes;
- alternative models of care that expand the role of non-medical healthcare professionals and carers to overcome a shortage of qualified healthcare professionals.

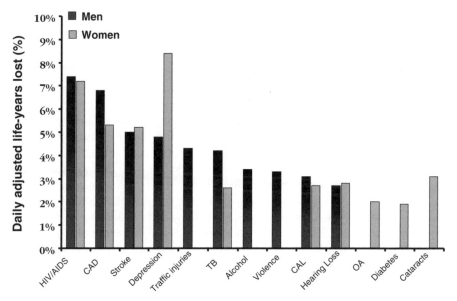

Figure 4.1. Conditions that have the greatest impact on global disability and premature mortality: a world of research still to complete!

Adapted from: World Health Organisation, Atlas of Heart Disease & Stroke, Chapter 13: Global burden of coronary heart disease. World Health Organisation, Geneva, 2005: www.who.int/cardiovascular_diseases/resources/atlas/en/print.html.

Most of the premier funding bodies in these countries (e.g. the National Institutes of Health in the USA and the National Health and Medical Research Council in Australia) clearly identify the highest research priorities and fund them accordingly. Not surprisingly, cardiovascular diseases (comprising diabetes, stroke and coronary artery disease), mental health (including depression) and respiratory disease (e.g. asthma in childhood and chronic airways limitation in older individuals) are typically high-profile conditions. In terms of the 'epidemiologic transition', there is also an emerging trend to suggest that the battle against chronic disease is being undermined by increasing rates of obesity, sedentary lifestyles and smoking in younger individuals. As such, there are fears that a second epidemic of cardio-respiratory disease will emerge in future generations without successful strategies and treatments to combat the same. Targeting this multifaceted phenomenon clearly represents a rich area of research for the foreseeable future.

In developing countries, there is a twin threat of infectious disease (e.g. HIV/AIDS and tuberculosis) and the emergence of 'Western' diseases due to the adoption of Western lifestyles. Research funding from the World Health Organisation and large philanthropic organisations (e.g. the Gates Foundation and the Wellcome Trust) in addition to specific overseas funding streams from the National Institutes of Health in the USA typically target the following:

- infectious disease prevention programmes;
- 'self-help'/capacity-building programmes to enable communities to solve and manage local healthcare issues;
- monitoring of the epidemiologic transition of disease within whole populations;
- culturally specific healthcare programmes.

While the above provides a broad overview of the type of research priorities around the globe and likely 'hot' topics for the foreseeable future, it doesn't provide any information on the most elusive and prized 'animal' in research: a unique study that will make a dramatic impact in the context of a 'hot' research topic health issue. Not surprisingly, the 'hotter' the topic, the greater the number of researchers and funding directed towards that field of endeavour. For example, consider the enormous amount of time and energy focussed on developing a cure for cancer or a vaccine for HIV. Consider also the accolades and rewards given to those researchers who achieve such seemingly impossible goals.

NEW RESEARCH HORIZONS: THE HEART OF SOWETO STUDY

One of the consistent themes in this book is taking a chance and making something out of what might have been nothing without your passion, input and willingness to gamble with your time and energy. As with the majority of exciting projects I've been involved with in my career thus far, the Heart of Soweto Study (described below and see Figure 4.2) began with a simple question from a mentor (Professor David Wilkinson, who was Pro Vice Chancellor of the Division of Health Sciences at the University of South Australia): *How would you like to travel to Johannesburg in South Africa to explore a potential research opportunity?* Although Professor Wilkinson was comfortable with the thought of travelling to South Africa, having spent a substantial portion of his clinical and research career there building programmes to combat AIDS and tuberculosis, I allowed my initial prejudices,

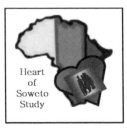

'Monitoring the pulse of South Africa's heart health'

THE HEART OF SOWETO STUDY

Professor Karen Sliwa, Witwatersrand University RSA
Professor Simon Stewart, Baker Heart Research Institute, Aus
Professor David Wilkinson, University of Queensland, Aus
Professor John McMurray, University of Glasgow, UK

Figure 4.2. The Heart of Soweto Study

formed by a seemingly unrelenting stream of unfavourable reports (both formal and informal) from developing countries on the African continent, to prevaricate in making any decision to join him. Fortunately, after some of my own homework and an inherent desire to seek out new research opportunities (wherever they lay), I travelled to Johannesburg and met a remarkable cardiologist (Professor Karen Sliwa) at one of the world's largest hospitals and the remarkable people and community of Soweto.

As with any collaboration, the Heart of Soweto Study has required an enormous amount of goodwill, give and take on both sides and perseverance to establish. This is typical of a long-distance, international collaboration that can quickly disintegrate through misunderstanding and an unequal power relationship (particularly if the 'host' researchers feel overpowered by the interests of the external partner). Notably, thus far, this project has thrived without competitive funding (an initial application for funding under the Wellcome Trust's populations in epidemiological transition funding scheme was rejected) and relied upon private funding sources (e.g. TigerBrand and Adcock Ingram in South Africa) that have recognised the enormous marketing/branding opportunities of the project when coupled with potential benefits for an internationally renowned community.

The following section, describing the rationale and activities (both past and proposed) relating to this study, is based on a recent application to extend the funding of the study through private sources. Hopefully, it conveys the passion, goodwill and momentum that form the basis of the best of collaborative research projects. Certainly, after the opportunity to present the progress and future of the study in a series of oral presentations, the study was granted further funding. Those aware of my own research interests will note that this study has all the *hallmarks* of my personal 'wish list' for a research project:

- focus on an important health issue: the global phenomenon of epidemiologic transition in developing countries;
- epidemiologic research related to cardiovascular health/disease;
- community engagement/empowerment;
- local capacity building.

BACKGROUND

Like many other parts of the globe, South Africa is experiencing a transition towards greater wealth and prosperity. With improved socio-economic conditions comes the opportunity to tackle key public health issues relating to improved law and order, with fewer accidental and violent deaths and better disease control to reduce the number of deaths caused by infectious disease. Improved economic conditions and the prospect of a longer life do not, however, come without a cost. As people live longer and adopt more affluent lifestyles, their risk of developing heart disease (a so-called 'affluent disease') dramatically *increases*. It has been estimated that within the next 20 years, 1.3 million people per year will be affected by heart disease in Africa.

Heart disease has the potential to not only cause disabling symptoms but also result in premature death in those who would have otherwise lived to old age. Fortunately, many of the causes of heart disease (e.g. high blood pressure, obesity, diabetes and smoking) are either treatable or completely preventable.

The key challenge for South Africa is to better understand the 'drivers' that are leading to the emergence of heart disease and to tackle them via better prevention and treatment programmes.

HEART DISEASE IN SOWETO

Established close to the city of Johannesburg, South Africa, 100 years ago, Soweto now represents one of the largest urban areas on the African continent. Home to more than one million people, the population of Soweto has benefited from improved economic conditions and public health advances in recent years. Unfortunately, the 'cost' of these improved conditions has been an increase in the number of individuals seeking medical care from the Cardiology Unit at the Baragwanath Hospital for heart disease or its common precursors.

For example, in the past 20 years, the number of people being treated for a heart attack in the Coronary Care Unit of the hospital has increased more than 10-fold and, in a typical clinic day, more than 100 people are seen in the outpatient clinic at the hospital for a heart-related condition.

THE HEART OF SOWETO STUDY

It was in response to the growing need for healthcare services for those affected by diseases of the heart that the Heart of Soweto Study officially began in January 2006, with key funding support from Unite 4 Health/Adcock Ingram.

Led by Professor Karen Sliwa (Director of the University of the Witwatersrand's Soweto Cardiovascular Research Unit at the Baragwanath Hospital), together with collaborating experts from Australia and the UK, the Heart of Soweto Study has begun the important task of better understanding and monitoring the emergence of heart disease in the local population and developing better healthcare services in response.

Mission Statement: The primary purpose of the '*Heart of Soweto Study*' is to *systematically* examine and respond to (with the creation of enhanced community health care services) the epidemiologic transition in risk behaviours and clinical presentations of heart disease in the predominantly black African population of approximately one million people living in the townships that comprise the internationally renowned and celebrated area of Soweto. In the process, the study team is committed to community engagement and building local research and health care service capacity.

This multi-phased project has a number of components that, when combined, are designed to reduce the burden imposed by the emergence of more affluent forms of heart disease in the local community. These activities include the following key phases of our unique and innovative programme:

Phase 1 Establishing a clinical registry of patients presenting to the Cardiology Unit at the Baragwanath Hospital.

Phase 2 Creating greater community *awareness* of heart failure in those at greater risk and provide more appropriate and culturally sensitive clinical services for those with heart failure in Soweto, with a strong focus on self-awareness/care.

Phase 3 Undertaking a community-based surveillance programme to better track and respond to the emergence of heart disease in Soweto.

WHAT WE HAVE ACHIEVED SO FAR!

Key activities undertaken as part of the initial stages of the Heart of Soweto Study have demonstrated our ability to build local research capacity and engage the local community and healthcare services in order to achieve our stated goals:

1. Tracking the emergence of heart disease! In addition to providing expert healthcare to those seeking treatment for heart-related conditions, the staff of the Cardiology Unit have established a unique clinical registry to describe each presenting case from the local population. *Since formally commencing this registry in early 2006, the study team have documented more than **3000 cases of heart disease** – the largest data collection of its kind in Africa.*

2. Improving outcomes in heart failure. One of the most debilitating and deadly forms of heart disease is heart failure: a condition that can occur following a seemingly normal pregnancy in young women or, more commonly, as a result of a heart attack or untreated high blood pressure in older people. *In order to improve outcomes in the increasing number of people affected by heart failure in Soweto (at least **600 heart failure patients/year**), the team have established a specialist heart failure clinic and links with the community to improve its management and typically poor health outcomes.*

3. Raising Heart Awareness in Soweto! With *Unite 4 Health/Adcock Ingram*'s support, each month, research nurses and doctors from the *Heart of Soweto Study* set up a 'screening station' within the community and provide free health checks for common risk factors for heart disease and healthcare advice or follow-up, if required. *With a target of 1000 participants, these 'Heart Awareness Days' have already discovered that **50%** of those screened have at least one risk factor for developing heart disease.*

The value of the vital research and community focus of the Heart of Soweto Study has been recognised by the enthusiasm of those working in the Soweto Cardiovascular Research Unit at the Baragwanath Hospital, the community

Number of admissions/million per annum

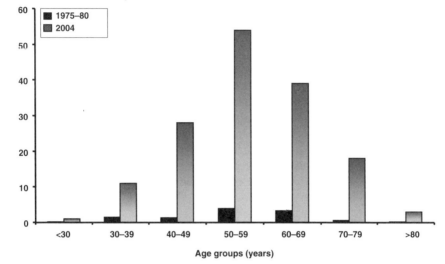

Figure 4.3. The number of cases of 'heart attack' being treated at the Coronary Care Unit of the Baragwanath Hospital over the past 30 years

of Soweto, the wider healthcare community and, indeed, international experts in the field, following the publication of a landmark paper describing the project:

Stewart S, Wilkinson D, Becker A, Askew D, Ntyintyane L, McMurray JJ and Sliwa K (2006) Mapping the emergence of heart disease in a black, urban population in Africa: The Heart of Soweto Study. *International Journal of Cardiology*, 108: 101–108

Consistent with the phenomenon of a community in transition from both a socio-economic and a health perspective, the Heart of Soweto Study has already uncovered a marked increase (more than 10-fold) in the number of cases of 'heart attack' being treated at the Coronary Care Unit of the Baragwanath Hospital over the past 30 years (see Figure 4.3).

INCREASING ADMISSIONS FOR HEART ATTACK IN SOWETO: A HISTORICAL COMPARISON

FUTURE ACTIVITIES

In order to build on the successful activities outlined above and provide a sustainable platform for the Heart of Soweto Study's role in monitoring and combating the inevitable rise in heart disease in the local community, it is vital that further funding is obtained to support three key areas of activity that directly relate to the three study phases outlined earlier in this document.

The *logical steps* arising from our initially successful programmes are the subject of our application for enhanced funding and relate to three key activities planned for the calendar year 2007, outlined below.

Phase 1	**Establish a clinical registry of patients presenting to the Cardiology Unit at the Baragwanath Hospital**
Extension:	**Proposed continuation of the Heart of Soweto Clinical Registry**

As described above, we have successfully established a 'Heart of Soweto Clinical Registry', documenting all clinical contacts in the newly renovated Baragwanath Cardiology Clinic since January 2006 (pilot data have been collected since October 2005). By the end of December 2006, we anticipate that this unique clinical registry will have collected the following clinical data:

1. the demographic profile and full spectrum of heart disease-related diagnoses of the approximately *3000 men and women* who have returned to the clinic for follow-up treatment in the year 2006 (*prevalent cases of heart disease*);
2. comprehensive demographic, cardiac risk, clinical and treatment data (including ECG and echocardiography) from the approximately *2000 men and women* who have presented to the Cardiology Unit (both the clinic and hospital wards) who have sought treatment for the *first time* in the year 2006 (*incident cases of heart disease*).

The *value* of these data cannot be overstated.

In just 12 months, it will represent the *largest clinical dataset on heart disease* emanating from the African continent. As such, it will provide an invaluable insight into the type and number of cases of heart disease arising from a predominantly black urban community undergoing significant socio-economic change.

Reports from this registry will be widely disseminated (including prestigious local and international conferences and medical journals) and used to inform decisions on how best to meet the needs of people who develop heart disease. The capacity building and information generated from our initial activities to establish this registry were instrumental in our successful attempts to implement 'Heart Awareness Days' in the local community (see below). In order to best understand the emergence of heart disease in Soweto over time, there is a logical need to systematically collect data over a prolonged period (i.e. beyond 2006). Having successfully established the clinical registry for patients with both pre-existing (so-called prevalence cases) and newly diagnosed (incident cases) heart disease, in addition to refurbishing the clinic at the Baragwanath Hospital to undertake this vitally important activity, there is a logical need to *extend data collection* to monitor potentially important changes in the following:

- number of new cases of heart disease presenting to the hospital: *Is it increasing each year or has the number of cases stabilised?*
- the pattern of underlying risk factors: *Are there more people with high blood pressure or diabetes?*
- the spectrum of heart disease: *Are there fewer 'infective' forms of heart disease and more 'affluent' forms over time?*

In order to address these key issues and questions, we propose to monitor all new cases (incident) of heart disease over the next calendar year (2007) in order to undertake important comparisons over the two-year period 2006 and 2007.

Phase 2	**Creating greater community *awareness* of heart failure in those at greater risk and provide more appropriate and culturally sensitive clinical services for those with heart failure in Soweto**
Extension	**Proposed establishment of a chronic heart failure awareness and management programme in Soweto**

It is important to re-emphasise that the increase in rates of coronary artery disease in Soweto does not appear to be confined to those presenting with an acute clinical problem (e.g. a heart attack). Our clinical registry has revealed that at least 20 per cent of new cases of heart disease presenting to the Cardiology Unit at the Baragwanath Hospital have developed CHF – a syndrome characterised by permanent structural or functional damage to the heart and accompanying neuro-hormonal and peripheral changes that leave affected individuals at greater risk of poor quality of life due to chronic shortness of breath, fatigue and peripheral oedema and a premature death. This equates to approximately *250 new cases of heart failure presenting to the clinic each year.*

Consistent with outcome data derived from patient cohorts in Western developed countries, 20 per cent of hospitalised patients with CHF at Baragwanath Hospital die within one year and 60 per cent of survivors are readmitted to hospital within 18 months. In the developed countries, there has been increasing interest in the role of dedicated CHF management programmes that provide individualised education, care and support to patients and families affected by this deadly and disabling syndrome. They have now become part of the gold-standard management of the syndrome. However, there are no data to support their use in a developing world context.

If better heart failure awareness and management are to be achieved in communities like Soweto, there has to be a strong community focus and use of available resources. It would be unsustainable, particularly given the natural focus on HIV/AIDS that has limited investment in tackling cardiovascular disease in South Africa, to establish the same kind of programmes that exist in developed countries. However, there are key components that could be adapted.

It is within this context and a careful analysis of the needs of the local community and the healthcare system to cope with an increasing burden imposed by heart failure that there is a clear need to undertake the following in Soweto:

1. raise the overall awareness of heart failure in those most at risk of developing this syndrome in Soweto;
2. establish culturally specific educational and support resources for patients and families affected by heart failure, with a strong focus on facilitating the self-care abilities of affected individuals to optimally manage their condition;
3. facilitate the optimal management of heart failure in Soweto by improving the local capacity of community-based nurses to manage patients and liaise with the expert heart-failure clinic located at Baragwanath Hospital.

In order to achieve these goals, we propose to establish a 'Chronic heart failure awareness and management program' in Soweto that will have *three* key features:

1. Development and distribution of a *CHF awareness brochure* that will be distributed to the thousands of patients attending primary care clinics in Soweto for any cardiovascular reason (including management of a risk factor, e.g. hypertension). The brochure will be designed to raise broad community awareness of the risk of developing this syndrome if common risk factors (including obesity and sedentary behaviour) are not addressed and to advise individuals when to seek appropriate healthcare if they develop symptoms indicative of the syndrome. The brochure will also be distributed at our regular community-based heart awareness programmes throughout Soweto.
2. Development and distribution of a *CHF patient support package* that will better enable the hundreds of affected patients to optimally *self-manage* their condition in the community.
3. Creation of a *nurse-facilitated, community-based CHF management programme* that integrates the currently fractionated care that patients receive from the Cardiology Unit at the Baragwanath Hospital and primary care clinics in Soweto to provide expert nursing and medical care across the whole continuum of the healthcare system.

Table 4.1. Summary of supplemental resource requirements and evaluation of outcomes to support the community, affected individuals and community nurses to improve health outcomes in relation to CHF

Program Activity	Resources	Evaluation
Raise overall awareness of CHF in high risk individuals attending primary care clinics in Soweto	Create and distribute easily understood (translations) CHF Awareness Brochure	Pre and post surveys to determine level of awareness of CHF and need to seek health advice when required Level of self-referral for potential CHF
Provide patients (and their families) with the necessary information and resources to optimally self-manage their CHF	Patient support package that include an individualised CHF self-care manual, key contacts and weigh scales (if required)	Patient/family awareness of the goals of optimal CHF management and level of self-care abilities to apply the best standard of management
Provide primary care nurses in Soweto with advanced training to best detect and manage CHF in the community	Appointment of 2 specialist CHF nurses to oversee this activity	Proportion of CHF patients on optimal management
Create better links between the Cardiology Unit at the Baragwanath Hospital with primary care clinics in Soweto via a nurse facilitated community management program	Provide regular training days and educational materials to nurses from 2 community clinics in Soweto Transport of nurses & patients to coordinate management	Rate of readmissions Survival Event-free survival Quality of life Health care costs Evaluation of *sustainability* of program

Table 4.1 summarises how the investment of funds to support this programme would be spent and subsequently *evaluated* in order to ensure that positive health outcomes are achieved.

If successful, this model of community engagement and specific integration of management will be extended beyond the two primary care clinics to be initially involved in the programme to encompass all primary care clinics in Soweto via funding applications to the South Africa government. Moreover, as 'proof of concept' is established, this model of care will be extended to other cardiac disease states and non-cardiac conditions.

Phase 3	**Undertake a community-based surveillance programme to better track and respond to the emergence of heart disease in Soweto**
Extension	**Proposed extension of the 'Heart Disease Awareness Days' to develop a systematic community screening programme**

In order to fully understand and respond to the 'drivers' of heart disease in Soweto, there is a clear need to move beyond those who present with pre-existing forms of heart disease to understand the following:

- What proportion of the local community are at risk of developing heart disease in the future because of pre-existing risk factors such as obesity, smoking, diabetes and high blood cholesterol levels secondary to a high-fat-content diet?
- What proportion of the local community have developed a non-symptomatic form of heart disease (i.e. they are unaware of their underlying disease) that will manifest itself in a potentially deadly symptomatic form over time?

At present, there are very limited data to answer either of these questions in *any* such community in other parts of the world, let alone Soweto. A natural extension of our successful 'Heart Awareness in Soweto Days' that will screen up to 1000 people by the end of 2006 is a more comprehensive and sophisticated examination of the risk factors and emergence of heart disease in the community. Such a programme would have the following features:

1. active screening of thousands of men and women from different parts of Soweto;
2. sophisticated but portable screening devices to examine heart and blood vessel function in addition to clinical and risk-factor data already gathered during the Heart Awareness Days;
3. assessment of dietary, exercise and other factors that may lead to the development of heart disease.

It is important to note that this activity will enable the team to evaluate the development of heart disease at a much earlier stage and plan for better 'primary prevention' strategies in Soweto while raising the awareness of the disease in the process.

SUMMARY OF PROPOSAL FOR SUSTAINED FUNDING

In the past 12 months (and, indeed, the preceding 12 months of planning), the Heart of Soweto Study research team has done much to understand the nature of emergent heart disease in Soweto and to determine the needs of those who are directly affected by it. However, much remains to be done and our efforts to establish the Heart of Soweto Study will have been in vain if we are unable to capitalise on the research capacity and infrastructure built on mutual cooperation and partnerships within the team itself and organisations such as Adcock Ingram/Unite 4 Health.

The planned activities for 2007 all represent logical extensions of the work that we have undertaken thus far. They have the potential to not only benefit the local community but also establish the study as an international exemplar for heart disease research in the developing world, particularly given the focus on developing culturally sensitive and sustainable community programmes to both prevent and treat heart disease effectively.

In the longer term, the research team believe that the growing spotlight on South Africa (and particularly Soweto, with its proud football heritage) for the 2010 FIFA World Championships will provide a fantastic opportunity to highlight the activities and sponsors of the Heart of Soweto Study. Securing funding for the next phase of the study's activities in 2007 will represent a fantastic platform towards securing the long-term future of the study and its presence in 2010.

TAKING IT ONE STEP FURTHER: IDENTIFYING A UNIQUE TOPIC

If anything, the Heart of Soweto Study demonstrates that there are still many opportunities to make a dramatic impact on health outcomes (around the globe) and build a successful research career as a result, particularly within the context of emerging health professions that have yet to explore their full potential and articulate the full extent of clinical areas of responsibility (e.g. the role of occupational therapists in disease management programmes for those with chronic cardiac disease). Identifying a unique contribution to health research overall and your health discipline is, therefore, still eminently feasible for novice researchers considering an academic career. There is no prescribed formula for discovering or identifying a unique research question or hypothesis to be explored and/or tested. Like most human activity, it can be derived from careful and strategic thinking and preliminary research or result from a moment of inspiration or consideration of an old problem in a new light. It is for this reason that the National Institutes of Health in the USA, for example, place such a strong emphasis on investigator-derived research (bottom-up) rather than a singular focus on prescribed research (top-down approach), although this is becoming increasingly more common globally with respect to funding translational research that bridges proof-of-concept to integration into the realms of health service treatment and delivery.

The first step, of course, is to recognise that the most successful researchers have built their careers on a seminal piece of research (usually early rather than later) by identifying or stumbling upon a unique research idea. Ultimately, finding an inspirational idea is most likely to happen when you are actively searching for it using a variety of methods. This can include:

- talking to mentors/role models about the potential areas of interest;
- reflecting on your own clinical practice;
- attending scientific meetings;
- carefully reading the literature around a particular topic;

- discussing clinical issues with your peers;
- considering parallel problems and solutions within other disciplines (e.g. education, information technology, psychology and business management).

Once you have identified a potential area of interest, it is important to determine whether any other research group or individual is examining the same area of research, but even if they are, you may well have the opportunity to improve on their ideas. Once again, this would involve attending scientific meetings relevant to the area of interest and undertaking careful literature reviews.

It is within this context that Figure 4.4 shows the inspiration and development behind my own evolving research programme focussed on nurse-led, multidisciplinary management programmes in patients with chronic disease, its evolution to a specific focus on chronic heart failure and a 'back to the future' focus on other forms of chronic cardiac disease. Remarkably, the inspiration for my research came from an educational psychologist who challenged me, during a graduate course that I was taking in adult education, to reconcile the practical implications of adult learning theory with the common practice of pre-discharge education of elderly patients (i.e. how well do we, as health professionals with expert skills and knowledge, prepare them to manage their own treatment and health on return to home). As can be appreciated from the course that I was taking, I was more interested, at that stage, in consolidating

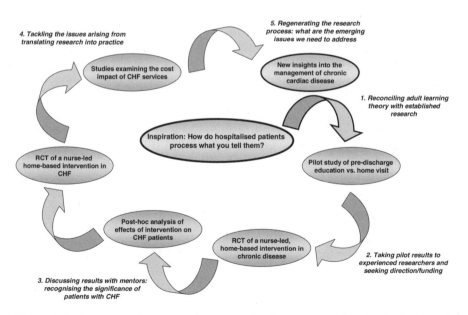

Figure 4.4. Anatomy of a research career: the importance of a single, insightful question!

a career in clinical education. However, his intriguing question led to me reading the literature, identifying a critical gap in what had been published and testing how well typically old and chronically ill patients remembered my talking to them about their medications in the hospital setting after one week at home. Much to my surprise, this simple study revealed that only one-third of patients remembered who I was, let alone remembered the information that I had given them during our lengthy session in the hospital! It was from this humble and inauspicious beginning that 'we' (I quickly realised that I needed expert help from experienced clinicians and researchers alike) ultimately designed a home-based management programme for patients with chronic heart failure, showing, for the first time ever, that such a programme could out-perform medical treatments with respect to prolonging the life of affected patients and dramatically reducing their rate of unplanned hospital stay.

If anything, Figure 4.4 is a classic example of initially 'thinking outside the square'. Although I can make no claim to the original, insightful question that led to my substantive research programme over more than a decade ago, I have certainly not underestimated the importance of looking beyond the embryonic discipline of nursing to generate research questions and clinical solutions. This is most definitely reflected in our development of a multidisciplinary model of care, rather than a singular intervention that exclusively focussed on the nurse–patient interaction. If you were to examine the early literature carefully in relation to heart failure management, for example, you might conclude that there was little room for more research. However, there are many individuals from a range of disciplines who are currently building strong research careers by exploring synergistic relationships between successful heart failure management programmes and more selective patient identification protocols, interventions (e.g. specific dietary plans) and surveillance systems (e.g. interactive monitors). Indeed, I am privileged to supervise a number of PhD candidates who have conveniently ignored my typical comments comprising 'so what' and 'oh please . . . not another heart failure study' to examine important issues with respect to optimising the application of dedicated management programmes; the specific details of two of these research programs – the BENCH Study and the CARDIAC-ARIA project – are outlined in a later chapter.

SUMMARY

The broad spectrum of healthcare issues that can be researched in order to improve health outcomes on an individual or population basis are, not surprisingly, enormous. In order to build a successful research career, however, it is important to focus on at least one major research area that, if you make a substantial contribution, will enable you to publish in high-quality/high-impact journals, engender interest from organising scientific committees of national and international conferences for invited presentations and, most importantly, will increase your chances of attracting sustained research funding. Choosing such a topic doesn't, in actual fact, preclude your spending your time and energy on much less fashionable research topics that give you the greatest satisfaction; it simply provides you with the opportunity to do so. Indeed, it is unwise to focus your energies in one particular direction. If you are too successful, you will research yourself out of a job! The process of identifying cutting-edge research and maintaining a healthy portfolio of research studies is one that should consume you for most of your research career.

Key Points: Unless you are content with small to modest funds to support your research, it is critically important to identify research topics that are likely to keep you at the forefront of 'cutting-edge' research for your discipline. Clearly, identifying health issues that have the greatest impact on whole populations and are the subject of 'priority' funding streams and high-profile research concentrations are the best place to start. However, it is still possible to make a successful career from a specialised issue, particularly if there is a 'knowledge/research gap' that clearly needs to be filled.

5 From Potential to Reality: The Importance of Achieving Timely Milestones to Bring your Research to Fruition

INTRODUCTION

It would appear obvious to anyone with a modicum of common sense that whilst identifying a 'hot' and potentially high-impact topic is an important start to a successful career, it is worth nothing if that potential is not brought to fruition through hard outcomes. In research, these outcomes include peer-reviewed publications, scholarships, research prizes, competitive grant funding and rapid career progression. As suggested in Figure 5.1, high achievers not only produce quality and quantity, but do so in a timely manner: many academics claim that they have published an impressive figure of more than 100 research papers, but if they have been researching for more than 10 or 20 years and have had the opportunity to build a large research team, a rate of 5–10 publications per annum is an under-achievement relative to opportunity! The concept of 'relative to opportunity' is particularly important when judging researchers in the early phases of their post-doctoral career, but does apply across the lifespan of a researcher. Accumulating an impressive curriculum vitae is about making every opportunity a winner. However, the squandering of potentially 'gilt-edged' research opportunities through the combination of any of the following is a universal phenomenon in the academic world:

- assuming that a brilliant research idea automatically equals a brilliant research study without proper planning and management strategies coupled with a personal commitment to hard work and critical thinking;
- under-estimating the capacity of other individuals and research groups to formulate the same research questions and then undertake the required research using a better study methodology and in a more timely manner;
- allowing critical phases of the research process (e.g. study design through to writing the major journal report) to be stalled through a lack of enthusiasm/team cohesion, leading to poor productivity or, paradoxically, allowing

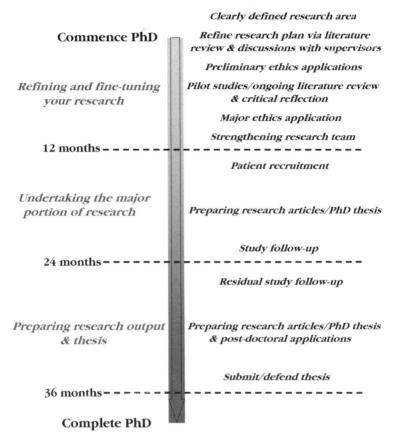

Figure 5.1. Mapping out a successful PhD

overly involved critical analysis and thinking to 'paralyse' the project into indecision;

• inadequate recognition of those key times when conflicting priorities are likely to impair your ability to commit to, and invest in, the research process;

• missing crucial dates when the impact of your research is likely to be at its highest (e.g. missing an abstract submission date for an international conference in your home country or not submitting a report to a specific issue on your topic of interest to a high-impact journal calling for papers on that particular topic).

In the absence of a reliable clairvoyant who can guide you through the process, it is often difficult to prospectively identify the specific landmarks that will increase your research impact and competitiveness. However, it still highly useful for you to map out the ideal progress of your research, with recognition of both positive and negative factors (as outlined in Figure 5.1), to identify how best the research question you've generated can be adequately examined and prepared for research presentation/publication and as evidence of rapid career progression. This is particularly important when your research forms the major portion of a PhD thesis – regardless of whether it is defended or presented in oral or written form.

COMPLETING A TIMELY AND SUCCESSFUL PhD

One of the most crucial components of a successful research career is *credibility*. It is not sufficient to call yourself a serious researcher without being able to back that statement with the credentials and qualifications that indicate that you have received appropriate research training from a well regarded institution and passed intensive internal and external reviews. Completing a timely and successful Doctor of Philosophy (PhD) or an equivalent qualification specifically related to a discipline and predominantly research-based (e.g. Doctor of Nursing Science – DNS) remains the *gold-standard* for gaining *initial* credibility as an independent researcher. Legitimately placing those magic three letters behind your name (remember that there are many apparently similar qualifications that are largely course-based rather than research-based) summarises a range of unique and advanced qualities that will immediately place you in the top tier of researchers. Unfortunately, many health professions remain in their infancy in terms of academic development and standards and are troubled by numerous 'teething' problems.

This problem is true of even the oldest of professions like nursing and midwifery and the issues that it currently faces in relation to offering quality research training is consistent with many non-medical professions that are yet to develop a consistent level of standards, the path of 'least resistance' and acceptance of mediocrity being a major hazard to the unwary, assuming that they are being prepared to the highest possible standards of research training. It should be noted that the following discussion in relation to the nursing profession is based on a published review of the same (Kirkman S, Thompson DR, Watson R, Stewart S, 2006).

THE ORIGINS OF ACADEMIC NURSING

Bachelor degrees in nursing and midwifery have only been available in the UK for approximately 50 years, pioneering university departments being Edinburgh, Manchester and Cardiff. From 2002 for midwives and 2004 for nurses, entry preparation below bachelor level has been discontinued in Wales, but diploma courses are still offered elsewhere in the UK. As the basic courses have evolved to graduate level, traditional nurse educators/academics have tried to keep at least one step ahead by obtaining post-registration bachelor degrees in the 1960s and 1970s, Masters degrees and, ultimately, PhDs in a range of health-related subjects.

Inevitably, as the tension for greater academic status has heightened, doctoral degrees have become more attractive to educators, clinicians and, indeed, a new generation of clinical researchers. Table 3.1 (see pages 32–36) shows that consistent with this observation, in terms of clinical research, post-doctoral applicants are still predominantly aged in their 30s or 40s in Australia. The number of those aged in their 20s (and presumably taking a direct path to research) is still relatively low. Unfortunately, at a time at which doctoral degrees have become increasingly important to the up-skilling and professional identity and academic integrity of the nursing profession, there is no consensus on what constitutes the best pathway to prepare for what should be an academically demanding and prestigious degree and, moreover, what form it should take.

It is important to note that in the absence of academic rigour and robust internal critique of clinical practice, professional knowledge and research, nursing and midwives and other health professions in a similar phase of 'academic development' are unlikely to be regarded by other professionals and health authorities as important 'players' in determining future health directions. At an academic level, initial tolerance of poor academic standards and output based on the 'infancy' of nursing and midwifery and other health professions at the tertiary level is likely to fade rapidly in the face of comparisons with other health professions who have managed to adopt the highest possible academic standards without compromising their unique identity and role in delivering healthcare.

It is within such an environment that the novice researcher should carefully consider the following questions in relation to the types of doctorates offered by the vast array of academic institutions:

1. Are all doctorates 'equal'?
2. If not, are some 'doctorates are more equal than others', despite apparent similarities and tendencies for the uninitiated and unwary to assume the former?

ESSENTIAL FEATURES OF THE DOCTORATE OF PHILOSOPHY (PhD)

Traditionally, any definition of a PhD contains the elements that a student will have carried out work which is independent, sustained, rigorous, original and at the cutting edge of the chosen field of research. It is also commonly expected that the researcher will demonstrate their competence as an independent researcher in a tangible way. In many countries, the examination of a PhD candidate is in one or two parts – a written and/or oral defence of PhD thesis. In Australia, for example, the oral defence has been largely dispensed with. In Europe, the defence of a PhD thesis by oral viva is a public event. However, it only enters this phase when the examiners are quite satisfied with the quality of the research being presented. In many institutions, provisional candidature is awarded as 'probationary' status until the candidate has provided evidence of their comprehensive understanding of their area of research and made strong progress towards preparing for their 'core' work towards the PhD; this may take anywhere between 6 and 12 months on a full-time basis. Where an oral examination is held, many universities are moving towards having the event overseen by an independent chairperson. In every case, at some point, the student registers their research proposal and has at least one academic supervisor. There can be more, but one person usually nominates to be the primary supervisor. In every case, if there is data collection emanating from human subjects, ethical approval must be sought and awarded.

VARIATIONS IN PhD PREPARATION

The 'traditional route' to a PhD has a surprisingly short history in the UK and other developed countries. For example, it was first approved by the UK Universities Conference in 1917 (Simpson 1983). The PhD candidate traditionally undertakes the equivalent of three or four years' full-time study and studies a subject in great depth, often carrying out empirical research involving data collection. In many disciplines, students are required to teach undergraduate students as a small but remunerated part of their work. The student meets their supervisor at intervals determined by them both, maybe only once a term, although there is increasing pressure by academic institutions worldwide to formalise the supervisory process. In some universities, therefore, both student and supervisor complete progress reports and there is often a formal transfer report which goes to a committee to approve the continuation of the study after about one year of full-time work. There may be a programme of research ongoing in the department and the student may take part in this, but his or her study must be independent. Exactly how this is achieved and which parts are then 'absorbed' by the candidate for their thesis research is the responsibility of the supervisor. External scrutiny of the proposal and of the transfer report is often sought to improve the academic rigour of the degree and associated research. During the last year of study, the supervisor makes arrangements for the appointment of examiners – usually one internal and one external. These examiners have to be approved by the university and they are paid for their work. The examiners read the thesis and then (in Europe and the USA at least) meet with the student at an oral examination. It has come to be seen as an essential research training to enable a graduate to enter his or her profession as a researcher.

   A significant variation from the 'traditional PhD' as outlined in the above paragraph is the 'taught doctorate'. This degree is most commonly found in the USA. In a marked departure from the 'free-form' PhD outlined above, the student enrols and commences a programme of taught modules in subjects focussed on teaching a person how to do research. These are subjects such as research methods, statistics, ethics and data analysis. The taught phase of the degree may last for one year or for as long as three years. Cohorts of students embark on their studies together, as this produces economies of scale for lecturing staff. Progress depends on the student's passing the modules. As the student cannot progress until a module has been passed, the course can take many years to complete. At a predetermined point, the student writes a research proposal, which is submitted to the faculty and, having been approved, the student embarks on a small project which may or may not include data collection. When the project is complete, it is examined and, along with the module results, a doctoral award is made.

Consistent with the modus operandi of a 'taught doctorate', the 'professional doctorate' is a major departure from the traditional PhD by research. In many cases, it can only be distinguished from the 'taught doctorate' on the basis of its title and relation to a specific discipline (e.g. Doctor of Psychology). Not surprisingly, it is not uncommon to hear that such degrees are the equivalent of a PhD without any substantiation for the same. Usually, the research and thesis component is considerably shorter than in a traditional PhD and it is hard to see how the same depth of argument can be sustained. Cohorts of students embark on the course together and accrue credits from the modules studied. The thesis is often professionally or practice based, focussing on an aspect of the student's professional scope of expertise and clinical practice. In some cases, such as clinical psychology, the doctorate has become the licence to practice (Hoddell 2000).

At the same end of the spectrum (closely linked to established knowledge and scope of practice) as the professional doctorate is the 'PhD by portfolio'. As part of this degree, the candidate submits written accounts of a number of different but related research projects that can be explicitly linked. As such, an over-arching statement of varying length (commonly 10,000 to 20,000 words) demonstrating any conceptual framework and showing how the projects are related to a whole are provided. Any publications arising from the projects can also be submitted (although this is more suited to the form of PhD detailed below). In many instances, the whole portfolio does not exceed the length (word count) of the traditional-route PhD for the host institution. Indeed, its aim is to be broadly comparable in depth and in breadth to the traditional-route PhD. Similarly to the professional doctorate, this degree ideally suits a person who has been in practice, rather than in academe, in a certain discipline and has built up his or her research expertise in an 'ad hoc' manner. A good example of its utility is given in the field of engineering, in which a graduate may have gone straight into practice and may have built bridges. To achieve this, he may have had to research new technology and brought together techniques in an innovative way, thus furthering his discipline by his actions. This degree offers practitioners the opportunity to show their contribution to knowledge. The portfolio of projects is examined in the same way as the traditional PhD.

More closely linked to the traditional PhD is the 'PhD by publication', but still consistent with the PhD by portfolio. In this form of PhD, the candidate submits a series of peer-reviewed, published papers that are linked by a clear theme. As such, an over-arching statement of up to 20,000 words demonstrating any conceptual framework and showing how the publications relate to each other accompanies these papers. The whole portfolio should not exceed the length (word count) of the traditional-route PhD for the host institution. Indeed, like the portfolio of projects route, its aim is to be broadly comparable in depth and in breadth to the traditional-route PhD. In the case of joint authorship, the candidate is asked to obtain written confirmation from the other author/s of his or her percentage contribution to the paper. This detail is closely scrutinised when the planned thesis is registered, not when it is submitted for examination. The portfolio of publications is examined in the same way as the traditional PhD. The role of the supervisor varies between institutions with regard to how detailed the accompanying statement is required to be (Powell 2004).

In any examination of the above forms of doctorate, it is worth considering some of the criteria outlined by the Quality Assurance Agency for Higher Education in the UK (published in November 2000) with respect to awarding doctoral degrees. As such, this report notes that doctorates are awarded to candidates who have demonstrated the following:

1. The creation and interpretation of new knowledge, through original research, or other advanced scholarship, of a quality to satisfy peer review, extend the forefront of the discipline, and merit publication.
2. A systematic acquisition and understanding on a substantial body of knowledge which is at the forefront of an academic discipline or area of professional practice.
3. The general ability to conceptualise, design and implement a project for the generation of new knowledge, applications or understanding at the forefront of the discipline, and to adjust the project design in the light of unforeseen problems.
4. A detailed understanding of applicable techniques for research and advanced academic enquiry.

As can be appreciated by the above summary of the different ways in which a doctorate can be attained, there are potential 'shortcuts' to such an award, but they may not be beneficial to your career in the longer term. Ultimately, any decision about what formal research training you receive should take into account what qualities you will develop at the end of the process. Typically, the harder and more high-powered environment you expose yourself to (i.e. a PhD in a world-class, research-intensive institution or group that only accepts the best from everyone), the better prepared you are to become an independent researcher in your own right.

KEY QUALITIES OF A PhD-QUALIFIED RESEARCHER

As indicated by the range of issues outlined above, it makes sense to carefully select the form of research training that you will undertake to emerge with the best possible array of skills and specialist knowledge. This section, therefore, focuses on the 'outcome' of your research training, as opposed to the way in which it is delivered. Not surprisingly, this particular section is prejudiced in favour of the traditional, free-form PhD, while acknowledging the various and more efficient ways (e.g. via the presentation of prospectively published series of articles) in which a PhD candidate can demonstrate that he or she deserves to be awarded the degree. It is within this context that it is worth considering the comprehensive list of attributes that have been articulated by the University of Melbourne (a research-intensive institution and regularly adjudged as being in the top 50 list of the world's best universities) with respect to those individuals talented and dedicated enough to complete a PhD (or equivalent). The following list certainly represents the high end of expectations for those entering the rarefied atmosphere of PhD-trained research, but why expect anything less?

- an advanced ability to initiate research and to formulate viable research questions;
- a demonstrated capacity to design, conduct and report sustained and original research;
- the capacity to contextualise research within an international corpus of specialist knowledge;
- an advanced ability to evaluate and synthesise research-based and scholarly literature;
- an advanced understanding of key disciplinary and multi-disciplinary norms and perspectives relevant to the field;
- highly developed problem-solving abilities and flexibility of approach;
- the ability to analyse critically within and across a changing disciplinary environment;
- the capacity to disseminate the results of research and scholarship by oral and written communication to a variety of audiences;
- a capacity to cooperate with and respect the contributions of fellow researchers and scholars;
- a profound respect for truth and intellectual integrity, and for the ethics of research and scholarship;
- an advanced facility in the management of information, including the application of computer systems and software where appropriate to the student's field of study;
- an understanding of the relevance and value of their research to national and international communities of scholars and collaborators;
- an awareness where appropriate of issues related to intellectual property management and the commercialisation of innovation; and

- an ability to formulate applications to relevant agencies, such as funding bodies and ethics committees. (www.ecom.unimelb.edu.au/future/pgrad/phd.html (accessed June 2005))

It is especially worth highlighting the statement of the need for graduates to possess 'a profound respect for truth and intellectual integrity'. This should not only relate to your external research activities, but also to your own capabilities as a researcher (i.e. have you taken the easy road to becoming a researcher via a lesser qualification or less stringent review process?) and how you present your qualifications and capabilities (i.e. misrepresent the importance of your research and/or your ability to undertake more advanced research). This obviously requires the kind of critical assessment outlined in Chapter 2. Considered in isolation, one could easily become overwhelmed by the list of graduate qualities outlined above. The same might be said of the extensive list of ancillary skills and knowledge domains also outlined in Chapter 2. However, if appropriately stimulating and challenging, your research training and miscellaneous experiences, combined with hard work and a determination to continually improve, are likely to provide you with the opportunities to develop these key graduate qualities, often without specifically addressing them. As noted in Chapter 1, it is imperative that your mentors/supervisors have a clear and impartial (other than wanting the best for you) understanding of what you need to succeed. They should also apply the principles underlying best practice in PhD supervision. This is particularly important in emerging health disciplines in which there is a general lack of research culture (Thompson DR, Kirkman S, Watson R, Stewart S, 2006).

Although completing a timely and successful PhD is not all about the written word or oral defence but more about the qualities that you develop, there are concrete milestones that are often used to determine whether you are setting a 'winning pattern' for long-term success early in your research career (see Figure 5.1). It is within this context that Figure 5.1 provides an example of the ideal milestones for a full-time PhD that has the following features:

- a strong preliminary plan for the topic of research prior to commencing enrolment;
- thorough and detailed planning and preparation in the first 12 months of enrolment, as demonstrated by a comprehensive and critical review of the literature, research team-building, pilot studies for determining the overall feasibility of the study with respect to patient recruitment, study follow-up, specific tools and questionnaires and clinical support, where required, in addition to the overall amount of time and energy required to complete the substantive research study/studies;
- early consideration of the overall focus and presentation of the PhD, with time set aside during routine research activities in years 2 and 3 to prepare for final presentation;
- an emphasis on publishing and preparing research papers early (i.e. review papers, pilot studies, rationale for study design, baseline characteristics,

major sub-studies and at least one major research report), as this allows for expert feedback beyond your immediate research team, provides you with a good sense of where your research sits internationally, as well as provides a strong reason why your PhD examiners should perceive your research as acceptable;

- time set aside for you to prepare a post-doctoral fellowship application in order to progress your research career further.

Within an overall strategic framework, it is possible to set firm milestones that take account of key dates for ethics, conference abstract submission deadlines, conference meetings and, importantly, personal commitments (e.g. Christmas holidays). A working example of the third year of a PhD candidature may include:

- 31 January – finalised Chapter 1 (subject review with copy of published review paper included in thesis), Chapter 2 (study design and rationale with copy of published paper) and Chapter 3 (pilot studies with copy of published research report);
- 28 February – recruitment of final study patient;
- 31 March – finalised Chapter 4 describing patients' characteristics and results of initial sub-study (research paper to be submitted to the *Journal of Advanced Journal of Nursing*);
- 10 May – submission of two research abstracts to International Conference on Chronic Disease Management;
- 30 June – submission of post-doctoral fellowship application;
- 31 September – complete follow-up of final patient (six months' follow-up);
- 15 December – finalise Chapter 5 (major study with submission of article for peer review to the *British Medical Journal* and secondary paper to *International Journal of Advanced Nursing* and Chapter 6 (summary chapter);
- 31 January – submit/defend complete PhD research programme.

With a prospectively designated PhD framework/research topic, it is much more feasible to reformulate milestones and/or plan accordingly for other research activities should unforeseen delays or problems occur. In most cases, it is extremely wise to formulate two alternative plans that will both result in your completing a timely and successful PhD. 'Plan A' usually represents the preferred option whereby there is competitive funding to support planned research and the likelihood of publishing reports in high-impact journals (see Chapter 6). 'Plan B' will usually represent a more 'realistic' option that takes into account the possible lack of funding, poor recruitment or publication of results from other sources that render your original research redundant. However, the alternative plan doesn't have to necessarily be inferior to the first and may, indeed, prove to be superior, particularly if it forces you and your supervisors/mentors to think more creatively. Figure 5.2 outlines a classical

Beyond city limits: Optimising the management of CHF patients in rural & remote Australia

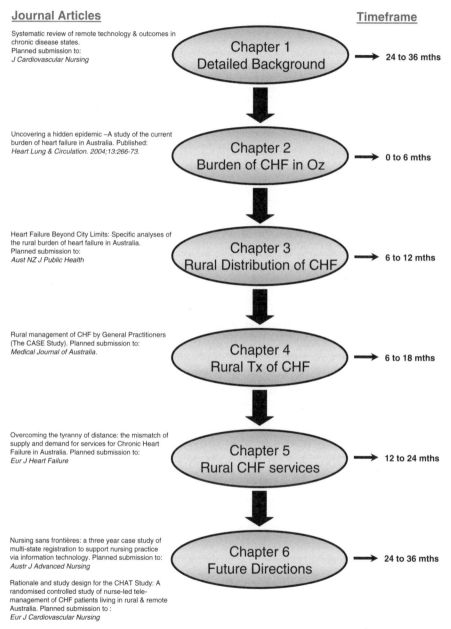

Journal Articles

Systematic review of remote technology & outcomes in chronic disease states.
Planned submission to:
J Cardiovascular Nursing

Uncovering a hidden epidemic –A study of the current burden of heart failure in Australia. Published:
Heart Lung & Circulation. 2004;13:266-73.

Heart Failure Beyond City Limits: Specific analyses of the rural burden of heart failure in Australia.
Planned submission to:
Aust NZ J Public Health

Rural management of CHF by General Practitioners (The CASE Study). Planned submission to:
Medical Journal of Australia.

Overcoming the tyranny of distance: the mismatch of supply and demand for services for Chronic Heart Failure in Australia. Planned submission to:
Eur J Heart Failure

Nursing sans frontières: a three year case study of multi-state registration to support nursing practice via information technology. Planned submission to:
Austr J Advanced Nursing

Rationale and study design for the CHAT Study: A randomised controlled study of nurse-led tele-management of CHF patients living in rural & remote Australia. Planned submission to :
Eur J Cardiovascular Nursing

Timeframe

Chapter 1
Detailed Background — 24 to 36 mths

Chapter 2
Burden of CHF in Oz — 0 to 6 mths

Chapter 3
Rural Distribution of CHF — 6 to 12 mths

Chapter 4
Rural Tx of CHF — 6 to 18 mths

Chapter 5
Rural CHF services — 12 to 24 mths

Chapter 6
Future Directions — 24 to 36 mths

Figure 5.2. Working example of a highly successful 'Plan B' PhD thesis

'Plan B' PhD in progress for Ms Robyn Clark – a National Institute of Clinical Studies and National Heart Foundation of Australia Postgraduate Research Scholar who, at the time of finalising this book, was a third-year PhD candidate at the University of South Australia, preparing to submit her thesis for examination. Initially, she was planning to base her PhD around a nationally competitive-funded project examining the benefits of a nurse-led telephonic support intervention for people with chronic heart failure living in rural and remote regions of Australia via a large cluster, randomised control trial involving more than 600 patients (the CHAT Study). Her major aim was to examine ways to optimise the management of chronic heart failure in patients living outside of the major healthcare networks currently established in Australia. Unfortunately, due to slow recruitment of patients via general practitioners in rural and remote Australia, the study is most likely to be completed beyond the target PhD completion date for Ms Clark. Therefore, rather than delay her PhD and her research career, we were able to carefully re-examine her specific research questions and the overall research topic to formulate a series of innovative studies that would (a) quantify the burden of heart failure in rural and remote Australia, (b) examine the current pattern of management via traditional sources of healthcare, (c) examine the penetration of specialist services into more remote regions of Australia, (d) explore the evidence base in favour of remote monitoring programmes in heart failure and (e) explore the potential impact of the CHAT Study and the types of practical/translational issues that will need to be addressed in the future. As can be appreciated by Figure 5.2, her PhD studies will still generate new research knowledge and are built on a series of peer-reviewed publications. As such, it will still form a strong basis for her post-doctoral research studies and complement the eventual completion and reporting of the CHAT Study. Indeed, the successfully funded research project CARDIAC-ARIA (original application presented later in this book) is an extension of her PhD research.

CONSOLIDATING A FOUNDATION FOR SUCCESS: POST-DOCTORAL FELLOWSHIP

Pointless as it may seem, it would appear that a large proportion of healthcare professionals who successfully complete a PhD melt back into their original clinical or educational practice without fully using the type of graduate qualities listed above to either improve clinical outcomes or their own career status. The reasons for this are undoubtedly complex, but may be explained by a combination of the following:

• a lack of vision beyond attaining a status symbol of achievement (i.e. being called Dr);
• reaching the peak of individual potential and desire and having nothing more to put into a research career;

- a lack of career options – this is where 'true' mentors and supervisors who assist your career progression are critically important;
- a lack of ability and productivity, as evidenced by a PhD characterised by poor supervision, lack of scientific rigour and quality, lackadaisical assessment from peer reviewers applying sub-standard criteria for acceptability (usually based on quantity not quality) and a paucity of meaningful outcomes (e.g. scientific presentations, publications, policy changes and evolution of clinical practice).

Unfortunately, the latter is particularly prevalent in many emerging health disciplines (e.g. nursing). As any successful career researcher will tell you, once you've climbed 'Everest' and completed your PhD, your natural euphoria and sense of accomplishment will rapidly expire to be replaced by a dawning realisation that there are many more peaks to climb beyond conquering a PhD! One of these is undertaking successful post-doctoral studies that will place you on the path to independently leading your own research group and mentoring emerging researchers in the future. Fortunately, if you are motivated enough to take the next step beyond a PhD and consolidate your research experience into a Post-Doctoral Fellowship, the strong work ethic and graduate qualities that characterise a successful PhD candidate will hold you in a good position to succeed thereafter.

What are the hallmarks of a successful Post-Doctoral Research Fellowship and what does it to take to increase the probability of selecting the right research group and research stream to exponentially improve your research profile, skills and productivity? It is, first, important to note that the same principles used to strategically plan a successful PhD noted in Chapter 1 and more specifically earlier in this chapter should be employed. However, unlike the usual situation in which, at the start of your PhD candidature, you are largely an unknown quantity with the potential to succeed, during the latter stages of your PhD, you should be in a position to leverage a post-doctoral position with a quality research group on the basis of concrete evidence of your future potential. Given the frenetic activity usually associated with completing a productive PhD, it makes perfect sense to organise the next phase of your research career long before you complete your PhD. This usually means strategically planning your next step in the first or second year of your PhD, making the appropriate contacts (preferably in person, during a visit to the department or during a scientific conference), negotiating the conditions under which you will be accepted and supported, and applying for competitive funding (if required) long before you commence finalising your PhD. Ideally, a successful post-doctoral position will have many of the following features:

- the opportunity to work with a truly international research team that it is totally distinct from the one that hosted your PhD;
- the opportunity for your research to naturally evolve into new areas (i.e. within the same discipline and focus but examining another important issue);

- the opportunity for personal growth in terms of new experiences, friendships, mentors, knowledge domains and skills;
- competitive funding with additional travel funds to facilitate conference attendance and visiting other research groups – it is always more attractive to your host and strategically helpful in negotiating exactly what research you want to perform if you are financially self-sufficient;
- high productivity in terms of presentations at international scientific meetings, peer-reviewed articles in high-impact journals and the opportunity to contribute to internationally distributed books by high-profile authors in the field;
- the establishment of a productive long-term collaboration with your post-doctoral research team.

Ideally, at the completion of a successful PhD and Post-Doctoral Fellowship, you will be in a perfect position to negotiate a more permanent research position at the institution of your choice, to establish your own research team/concentration, either within an established team with access to more senior and experienced researchers or as a completely new entity. Having experienced the latter (i.e. attempting to build a completely new research team from nothing), I would personally advocate strategically placing yourself in an established research concentration with all its inherent advantages for immediate research success. The post-doctoral researchers profiled in Table 3.1 clearly recognise the value of competing for post-doctoral research support. Although many of these researchers would be disappointed by the results of peer review (remembering that there is a stated aim to support the most outstanding individuals), a large majority will be employed through other funding mechanisms (e.g. specific project funds).

Regardless of your ultimate research path, it is highly advantageous to bring an 'active collaboration' with your post-doctoral colleagues to the next phase of your research career. As will be discussed in the next chapter, in order to maintain research output and a high profile during naturally sub-optimal periods of research productivity (i.e. when you are in transition from one position to the other), it is extremely useful to have a productive collaboration and high-profile association with a research team that does not require your personal presence and input. Ultimately, your post-doctoral research studies should be productive enough for you to successfully launch the next phase of your research career without having to lose any momentum.

SUMMARY

Without a structured and strategically planned PhD and Post-Doctoral Fellowship that are completed in a timely manner and are associated with high productivity, it is very unlikely that you will be able to successfully compete for competitive research grants and therefore successfully apply for high-level research positions in the future. These critical phases in your research career set a pattern both in terms of your personal attributes and qualities and external perceptions of your strengths and weaknesses as documented in your curriculum vitae. With very few exceptions, highly successful researchers establish their credibility and quality in the early phases of their career. As noted throughout this book, they create a self-fulfilling prophecy for future career success.

Key Points: Your PhD and post-doctoral studies represent critical phases in your research career. Quite simply, they can make or break your future aspirations. A PhD cannot be considered in isolation. It has to be linked to a successful post-doctoral phase in a different institution with a different research agenda. Similarly, your post-doctoral studies have to be linked to your long-term plans to carve out your own research agenda and career. In research, there is no one single mountain to climb, but merely a series of peaks that inevitably lead to another challenging climb. As such, it is not for the faint-hearted!

---

6 Becoming a Prolific Publisher

INTRODUCTION

In the increasingly competitive world of academia, the mantra 'publish or perish' is becoming louder each year. The reasons for this are simple. Whether you are working in an academic institution located in the USA, Europe or Australasia, there is an underlying expectation that you will contribute to the overall productivity of the institution by publishing peer-reviewed research articles, invited articles, book chapters and even books (like this one!). Nearly all institutions and individual faculties rely on such productivity to not only demonstrate their contribution to a particular discipline or field of endeavour to external agencies, but also use it to leverage additional external funding relative to other institutions, in terms of both quantity and quality (i.e. as a demonstration of either a preponderance of national as opposed to international experts concentrated within that institution). Given that most institutions contain a blend of academics that vary in terms of the spectrum of educational and research activities that they undertake, it is generally accepted that a *minority* of highly productive academics will push the average number of research or scholarly publications per employed academic beyond the almost universal target of one peer-reviewed paper per year. These rare academics, therefore, not only 'feed' their own curriculum vitae and justify their existence through their academic output, but also 'feed' the institution's profile and assist in generating research incomes beyond the cost of their own salary.

In research-only institutions that contain a predominance of academics funded by competitive research grants, this standard figure may be much higher and also involve additional pressure to publish in high-impact journals (a description of what this actually means is provided in the text box). However, as noted at the beginning of this book, the emerging academic health disciplines (e.g. the nursing profession) as a whole has a poor record in generating scholarly reports based on their clinical practice and professional knowledge relative to other disciplines (most notably medicine). For example, such a record is reflected in the poor rates of publications per nursing academic in all developed countries, with only a few exceptions to the rule. It is also reflected in the nursing journals that have 'low' impact scores which do not mean that they are not read by many, but that they are not used and referenced by many other nurse clinicians or academics, or indeed, other health professionals, in generating and reporting on new research projects.

Regardless of the underlying cause of poor publication records endemic for nearly all healthcare-related disciplines, it is obvious that institutions around the globe highly value academics who can produce the goods in terms of regular publications, particularly if they appear in international professional journals or high-impact bio-medical journals that have the potential to influence clinical practice or scholarly thought around a particular health issue. Becoming a prolific publisher is, therefore, desirable to not only demonstrate your mastery of a particular subject, but also to increase the competition for your services.

ISI Journal Impact Factors: A journal's impact factor is a measure of the frequency with which their 'average' published article has been cited in a particular year or period. Monitored and published in journal ranking reports for various disciplines, the impact factor is useful in clarifying the significance of absolute (or total) citation frequencies. It eliminates some of the bias of such counts which favours high volume, generalist journals over small, more specialised journals. In terms of evaluating the relative worth of published research and academic status, the impact factor can be used to provide a general (but not absolute!) approximation of the prestige of journals in which individuals have been published. (ISI = Institute for Scientific Information; for more information, see www.isinet.com/essays/journalcitationreports/7.html/).

PUBLISHING: WHAT SHOULD YOU BE AIMING FOR?

As with most aspects of your academic career, publishing is not simply about the number of publications. It is also about the quality of journals, publishers and collaborators whom you work with and also the impact that your research and thoughts have on clinical practice and other healthcare researchers. In critiquing your own curriculum vitae, you should be examining the following three critical aspects of your publication record:

1. average number of publications per annum relative to the stage of my research career;
2. impact factors of the journals that I've published in and/or quality of journals relevant to my particular discipline area (e.g. midwifery as opposed to cardiovascular nursing);
3. number of citations of my papers by other academics subsequently publishing their own research or scholarly opinions or dissertations.

Rest assured that these are the same three measures that your institution, more competitive peers and/or external examiners for research scholarships and grants will use to judge your relative worth and productivity!

Rather than focus on any one particular area (i.e. produce one paper that appears in the *New England Journal of Medicine* with an ISI impact factor of around 27 as opposed to the one published in *Journal of Advanced Nursing* representing probably 1/2000th of the impact with an ISI impact factor of around 1.0), it is wise to aim for a *balanced* portfolio of publications that will appear to contain both quantity and quality to the external observer.

It is important to note that your productivity is inexorably linked to the stage of your research career and relative opportunity to publish original research (e.g. once you've completed a full-time PhD). Unless you belong to an international research team that will provide you with an endless supply of quality research papers for minimum effort to attain legitimate authorship (I'm yet to meet that lucky non-medical scholar!), you will have to be content with the cyclical nature of research output until you can form your own stable of researchers who provide a 'steady-state' of publications, with you as senior author.

Figure 6.1 tracks my own publication record, from the completion of my PhD in early 1999 to 2006, noting the number of publications, the total impact scores of journals in which they appear (as a reference, the *British Medical*

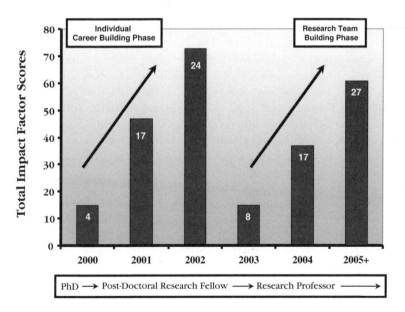

Figure 6.1. The inevitable peaks and troughs of publishing whilst building a research career: a real-life example

Legend: Number of peer-reviewed publications (white numbers within bars)

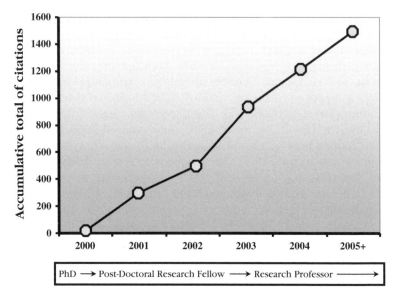

Figure 6.2. Monitoring the number of citations to your publications: an index of the real impact of your research

Journal had an ISI impact factor of around 5.0 for a number of years and is now around 9.0) and the progression of my role from post-doctoral fellow to a full-time Professor of Research. This type of analysis (whilst delivering a brutal message!) provides a clear insight into the cyclical nature of research; rest assured, I had few publications during my PhD. More encouraging is a graph showing the accumulated total of citations from your research reports, particularly if they are published in high-impact journals. Any paper that is cited more than 10 times within a few years of publication should be considered a success, with those approaching 50 citations highly successful and more than 100 citations approaching a 'seminal' contribution to the literature. Figure 6.2 provides an approximation of my citation record over the last seven years (i.e. since completing a PhD); naturally, given the accumulative figures, it looks much more reassuring than the cyclical nature of annual publications. As an individual researcher relying on my own PhD research, I was able to publish six papers in 1999 and four more in the year 2000, the most notable being a report on a randomised–controlled trial of a nurse-led intervention for patients with chronic heart failure, published in *The Lancet* in 1999 (with a very high ISI impact factor score). Naturally, this particular paper inflated my 'impact factor score' for 1999 and provided me with the momentum to gain an overseas post-doctoral research fellowship. As a result, I was more than fortunate to work with an internationally renowned research group led by Professor John McMurray at the University of Glasgow, who provided me with the opportunity to publish a large number of research papers over a frenetic two-year period (2001/02). My publication record in 2003 (my first full year as a research professor) is a sobering reminder of what happens when the amount of research material that you have to publish with, and collaborative researchers whom you have to work alongside, suddenly subsides! Thanks to residual links to my post-doctoral colleagues, I was able to maintain a reasonable publication record in 2003. By 2004, my attempts to generate new research data and build a research team comprising PhD candidates and post-doctoral fellows, in addition to strengthening links to other researchers, appeared to have had a positive impact on my publication record. The challenge, of course, is to maintain a reasonable record: my research team now aims to publish 20 peer-reviewed papers per annum, with a combined impact factor equivalent to three to six *British Medical Journal* papers each year.

If this graph and personal 'publication biography' tell you anything, it is that your own publication target should reflect the stage of your career. For all of my PhD candidates, I advise the following in terms of publication output:

1. Publish at least five research reports from your PhD – the higher the impact factor, the better, but this will, of course, depend on your research subject (see Chapter 4).
2. Target a highly productive research team for your post-doctoral research training in order to gain both team publications in high-impact journals that require minimal effort and a wealth of research data to write as many of your own publications as possible. You should aim for a research team that will give you the potential to publish at least 10 research papers per annum.
3. Even when you are in a building or rebuilding phase of your research career, you should aim for at least five publications per annum.

The third target necessitates planning as soon as possible for the 'lean' years, when you are rebuilding your publication potential, by making the effort to maintain good relationships with your mentors (e.g. PhD supervisors and post-doctoral hosts) and other researchers willing to collaborate to enhance their own publication output. As I'm in the process of rebuilding a team, my own target will prove to be a challenge, but hopefully not as onerous as the last time (2003) given a larger 'residual' group of researchers and PhD collaborators with whom I'm able to generate data and publish quality research reports.

KEY ATTRIBUTES OF A PROLIFIC PUBLISHER

Becoming a prolific publisher requires two simple ingredients, both of which usually require hard work, dedication and strategic planning. The first of these is excellent writing skills. Excellent writers use a minimum of words to convey complex ideas and vivid images. Almost everyone has their own idea of how these might be conveyed. However, a good writer is able to please a large number of people without receiving a plethora of editing comments. In all honesty, I still cringe when I receive the electronic 'red deletions' indicative of electronic track changes in a Word document as a hangover of my torment at the end of the red or green pen of my PhD supervisor, Professor John Horowitz, in South Australia and my post-doctoral host, Professor John McMurray, in Scotland! Very few people possess the ability to write and convey ideas elegantly and succinctly without years and years of practice; rest assured, this book has been heavily edited by a dedicated editor employed by the publisher! Most serious researchers will tell you that they have a surplus of research data but a dearth of writers who have both mastery of the subject and the ability to write an excellent manuscript requiring minimal editing. Prove yourself to be a good writer who can turn data into publishable material and you will be in high demand by the very best researchers.

As always, practice makes perfect, and improving your writing skills via the following strategies is highly recommended:

- working regularly with expert writers (preferably your PhD supervisor and/ or other mentors will be prolific publishers with excellent skills) who will be exemplars of good writing;
- reading both good and bad books/articles, taking formal writing courses and using the services of dedicated editors (many academic departments employ such individuals);
- attempting to write in different styles (i.e. a comprehensive review versus pure scientific report on a specific research study);
- exposing your writing to critical review as early as possible in your research career via peer-reviewed journals;
- examining more than one way to publish (i.e. offering to write book chapters and books with more experienced colleagues).

There is a natural tendency to assume that once you've mastered one significant writing test that has passed public scrutiny (for many people, it is their PhD thesis), you have reached the peak of your writing powers. Happily, this couldn't be further from the truth! Many experienced researchers are unable to read their earlier research reports without finding many faults. Writing, as with many skills, is a developing one that can only get better with practice, critical scrutiny, more practice and more critical scrutiny.

The second essential ingredient is, of course, a wealth of quality research material that will convince journal editors and peer reviewers that your submitted material is not only well written and presented, but adds something of significance to the literature. As indicated above, this requires careful strategic planning to ensure that you not only research in an area of national and, preferably, international significance, but collaborate with experienced researchers who have a large body of research that requires someone with excellent writing skills to produce the final product.

In addition to the above, prolific publishers are always looking at ways to produce new research papers. Whilst this may appear obvious, it takes a certain mindset and determination to take advantage of every opportunity to publish; I particularly admire my friend and mentor, Professor David Wilkinson from the University of Queensland, for examining every opportunity to publish and making it happen. For example, the time and effort to prepare a comprehensive literature review for a grant application (see Chapter 7) represent a perfect opportunity to prepare a comprehensive review article. They also take careful note of the various requirements and styles requested by journals and publishers; remember, with a surfeit of written material, editors are likely to 'default' papers submitted with the wrong formatting and/or poor spelling/grammar. If a paper has been accepted in a particular journal, it will undoubtedly have qualities (e.g. style of writing) that can be readily adopted to improve your own paper. Prolific publishers also pay close attention to the overall presentation of their submission, with the use of bold and innovative graphics and simple but striking formatting. They also take careful note of the feedback provided by editors and peer reviewers, take the time to address specific points and provide a balanced response; why pick an intellectual argument with those with the power to decide the ultimate fate of your article, chapter or book?

As indicated above, publishing is not only just about peer-reviewed journals in high-impact journals; it is also about the following:

- published abstracts from scientific meetings involving merit selection via peer review;
- research monologues published via your academic institution;
- official reports emanating from contracted research;
- book chapters;
- edited books (i.e. where you act as the editor and coordinate and edit the content written by a panel of researchers/writers);
- research-only books based on your area of expertise – given some formatting, a clinically relevant PhD with a logical flow comprising a comprehensive literature review, ground-breaking research and a summary of the clinical implications/translation to healthcare treatments/services is likely to be publishable (this is a practice already inherent to many PhD candidates from European institutions who fund their own publication of their thesis).

Taken together, all of the above provide a rich fabric of research output and are attainable by most researchers. As such, they are best facilitated by an experienced researcher/research team with a good track record in submitting scientific abstracts and obtaining publishing contracts. Once again, the demand for effective writers who are able to complete chapter and book contributions on time is extremely high – the ability to communicate effectively is prized as highly as effective research skills.

SUMMARY

One of the key characteristics of any successful academic researcher is a prolific publishing record. If you operate within a discipline with routinely poor publishing records, then becoming a prolific publisher will put you in high demand from institutions wishing to increase publishing rates within that discipline. A PhD should provide a wealth of opportunity to publish (at least five publications) and post-doctoral training even more so (at least 10 publications per annum). Early strategic intent and dedication to develop excellent writing skills and a wealth of research material are a prerequisite to a sustained publication output. Such an output will typically encompass both quality and quantity.

Key Points: Regularly publishing research papers in the highest possible impact journals is a major indicator of your worth to an academic institution and your overall standing within your discipline. Developing excellent writing skills is a critical and therefore non-negotiable part of being a successful health researcher.

---

7 Successfully Applying for Competitive Research Funds to Support your Career Path and Research Programme

INTRODUCTION

The 'oxygen' that drives a successful research career is ultimately competitive research funding. Unless you have an unlimited supply of personal research funds, your designated research programme and, indeed, competitiveness for more advanced academic/research positions will quickly stall without a steady supply of national and internationally competitive research funds. Like publishing, your relative merit to an academic institution is inexorably linked to your ability to attract competitive research funding in greater amounts than any of your immediate peers. Usually, for every competitive dollar/pound sterling/Euro you attract, your institution will usually receive additional funding and will always bask in the associated prestige. If you are fortunate enough to live in countries like the USA or Canada, you will most probably have access to dedicated funds for non-medical health disciplines. In these countries, the average level of research funds may be relatively high and you will have to work harder to 'overachieve' relative to your peers. In other countries, there may be a dearth of specific funding (e.g. Australia, where there is an 'unhealthy' imbalance favouring medical and basic research) for your discipline and any competitive funding success may be viewed favourably. Regardless of the environment in which you operate, however, it should be a career-long mission to apply for and obtain competitive research funding; some invoke the analogy of the greyhound endlessly chasing the 'rabbit', with little reward but much effort.

The following forms of research support are essential at critical phases of your career and, if successfully added to your curriculum vitae in a consistent and progressive manner, will make the job of attracting competitive funding support for each subsequent phase of your research career and research programme that much easier:

- post-graduate research scholarship to support a full-time PhD;
- post-doctoral research fellowship to undertake further research training with another research team within your home country, or more strategically for the longer-term with an internationally renowned and productive research team overseas;
- specific project funding for individual research studies; this will often include provision for 'new investigator' grants for researchers aiming to start their own programme of research;
- strategic research funding to support a research concentration and a team of researchers at various stages of their research career;
- specific funding for a systematic programme of research.

Clearly, the success of any application for personal support or project funding relies upon the strength of your curriculum vitae in addition to the quality and potential impact of the proposed research: the range of strategies outlined in previous chapters will all have a positive impact in this regard. However, your application for funding, no matter how good, is likely to founder unless it is presented in the best possible way. The following sections outline what you can do to impress your peers and compel them to fund your research activities, a major caveat being that every researcher, irrespective of their seniority, is fallible and likely to experience the bitter taste of rejection when competing for limited funding and so many health priorities.

IMPROVING YOUR CHANCES OF FUNDING SUCCESS

Before attempting to present your research (or personal credentials if applying for a research scholarship), what are the strategies that will improve your chances of gaining research funding even prior to constructing an application? Incorporating many of the strategies outlined previously, it is important to consider the following:

- Select a 'hot' research topic, particularly one that matches the funding body and is consistent with what they are likely to fund or support. As always, this requires advanced research to determine previously funded grants or researchers, seeking specific advice or information from the granting organisation or previous winners and adapting your research application accordingly.
- Publish your research whenever possible in high-impact, professionally important journals – particularly that arising out of competitive research funding. This clearly establishes your ability to complete funded research and produce quality reports that have the potential to make a substantial impact on health outcomes (see below).
- Wherever possible, attempt to translate your research into real life via policy documents, clinical guidelines, clinical practice and, if appropriate, healthcare services.

- Carefully select your research team (regardless of whether you are applying for a scholarship or a research grant) to first ensure that all the areas of research expertise that you require are covered (e.g. a health economist if undertaking a cost–benefit analysis) and, secondly, include a senior researcher who will provide the experience and expertise to both improve your research proposal and provide further guarantee to the assessors that the research can be completed successfully.
- Time your research and publication efforts to 'peak' around the time of the funding application to maximise your curriculum vitae.
- Undertake, present and publish comprehensive literature reviews and pilot research projects that support the hypotheses and research questions underlying your research. Consistent with the underlying philosophy of this book (a self-fulfilling prophecy), referencing your own article, indicating the need to undertake the same research as you are proposing, is particularly effective.
- Prepare and maintain the best possible curriculum vitae to highlight your key attributes and strengths. This is particularly important when preparing applications for personal support. It is also important when collaborating with other researchers to ensure that their curriculum vitae doesn't 'drag' the impact of other curricula vitae down through sloppy presentation. The importance of a visually appealing curriculum vitae is discussed in more detail in the next section of this chapter.
- Give yourself the maximal amount of time to prepare an application; in some cases, this is impossible due to unexpected calls for research applications. However, you should construct a research calendar for all the 'usual suspects' for research funding and plan your year accordingly.
- As indicated above, regardless of the merit of your research and quality of your track record, there is always likely to be an excess of applications and therefore strong competition for a limited amount of funding. The assessment panel will, therefore, be seeking easy ways to trim the list of competitive applications. Moreover, they and any peer reviewers will undoubtedly be suffering from 'reviewer fatigue' and will react negatively to poorly written applications or boring presentations. What are the hallmarks of an effective research application? Fortunately, there are many books that specifically cover this subject and represent a small investment of time and money relative to the opportunity to gain the critical edge in getting your research funded. Overall, an effective written application has the following features that will both satisfy and stimulate peer reviewers and highlight the best features of your research:
  - conforms with written instructions relating to structure, length, font size and use of graphics;
  - a focus on quality rather than quantity;
  - regardless of formal structural requirements, is clearly partitioned to include the rationale for the research, its overall significance to the discipline and overall health outcomes, the underlying hypotheses/research

questions, specific methods with commentaries on the feasibility, validity and reasons for the chosen methodology (e.g. justifying a nested, case–control study and not a prospective randomised controlled trial) in addition to including study power calculations, where appropriate, and, finally, a clear statement on why the proposal is so important in terms of improving health outcomes;

- contemporary references that indicate awareness of the latest research and its implications;
- good grammar, clear and concise concepts, no obvious spelling mistakes and readable font size – one of the easiest ways to attract a negative review is to make it difficult for a reviewer to read and understand the application!
- reinforcement of key points;
- clear and precise figures.

In the usual headlong rush to construct a research application, there is often little consideration of the need for an external reviewer to identify minor mistakes and, more importantly, identify/clarify issues that a formal peer reviewer would also target and potentially use to reject the application. For example, in a recent grant application for a national, multi-centre study of chronic heart failure management, my collaborative research team failed to identify a critical but very simple spelling mistake (a 'with' rather than 'without' was included) in our inclusion criteria that completely changed the tone of the research proposal. This simple mistake led the peer reviewers to question the entire purpose of the project and it was ultimately unsuccessful for funding. In the cruel world of competitive research funding, it is often one minor mistake that will undo months of planning and effort! As indicated above, it is imperative to give yourself time to plan your application with meticulous detail and allow for external reviews to identify even the smallest mistakes.

A key feature of readable and often successful research applications is clear and precise figures that convey or reinforce an important message or point without the clutter of words. Figure 7.1 demonstrates how you can convey

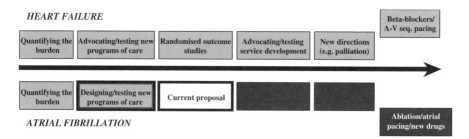

Figure 7.1. Placing your research in the context of what you have achieved and what you hope to achieve in a relatively simple graph

your substantive research and impact in one area (the top panel relating to heart failure) and how a new area of research (in this case, atrial fibrillation, as represented in the bottom panel) will be similarly developed via successful funding of your proposal.

PUTTING IT ALL TOGETHER AS PART OF A PERSUASIVE RESEARCH APPLICATION

As stressed in the introduction to this chapter, the 'oxygen' that drives a successful research career is, ultimately, competitive research funding and this obviously relies upon a persuasive research application. Consistent with a 'warts and all' approach to my own research, this section of the chapter provides details of two successful and one pending (having been short-listed for more intensive scrutiny) funding applications that are intimately linked. For example, the first successfully funded application presented below (for a very modest amount of AU$24,000 over 12 months, equivalent to £10,000 or €12,000), which was the focus of one person's PhD research (Ms Andrea Driscoll from Deakin University in Melbourne, Australia), was then combined with another person's PhD research (Ms Robyn Clark from the University of South Australia in Adelaide, Australia – see Chapter 5 for her PhD plan) to develop a completely new and innovative project worth more than AU$650,000 (equivalent to £250,000 or €325,000) over three years. The third and final application presented has used data from the first study to identify a key clinical/consumer issue to be addressed and provided a sound basis for why it can be undertaken in a timely manner.

Consistent with the amount of funding gained, the first project, named the BENCH Study, was successfully won from the modestly funded National Heart Foundation of Australia Research Grants-in-Aid Scheme that, at the time of its award, combined written applications subject to external expert peer review with interviews of potentially fundable applicants. This form of specific funding is *perfect* for a project that combines the generation of new knowledge in a specialty area (i.e. pilot research that is not yet ready for a major funding grant with competition from many health priority areas) and supporting a new investigator at the very beginning of their career who was able to be nominated as the Chief Investigator with the support of more senior colleagues. The BENCH Study (now in its final phases of activity and involving close to 1500 heart failure patients from more than 50 heart failure management programmes around Australia) has actually belied its modest funding status and generated a significant amount of data on heart failure management in Australia and led to other projects, including the CARDIAC-ARIA project and WHICH? Trial, described below.

The second project, therefore – CARDIAC-ARIA – with its much more substantive budget and complexity of research, was competitive for a number of reasons, not least because of the data generated from the modestly funded BENCH Study and its provision of data that provided 'proof of concept' for the innovative geo-mapping of cardiac services in Australia. The fact that CARDIAC-ARIA is being funded by the Australian Research Council's Linkage Grant Scheme (see specific details below) is especially notable given its focus on funding research proposals that are not normally covered by the Australian Health and Medical Research Council and combine partnerships between academic institutions and private industry.

The third and final project presented below – the WHICH? Trial – is a multi-centre trial of different forms of heart failure management and involving major collaborators strengthened through those links built around the BENCH Study. With a funding budget of around AU$900,000, it represents a quantum leap forward from the BENCH Study and will obviously provide an excellent framework for PhD and post-doctoral researchers, via funding from Australia's peak health research organisation – the National Health and Medical Research Council of Australia.

In presenting the substantive portions of each of these applications (remembering that most researchers have a *negative* record of applications that vary from 10 to 50 per cent, depending on their expertise and luck!), it is hoped that the reader will refer to the above section outlining the principles for success and make their own mind up in terms of whether (a) it should (have) been funded, (b) it could have been improved or (c) it's perfect! In mine and my colleagues' defence, I would reiterate that research and all its related activities are a life-long learning process. As with all of my past writing attempts, it is painful to identify obvious areas for improvement. External and critical self-critique is the obvious way to steadily improve key activities such as competitive grants applications.

APPLICATION 1: NATIONAL BENCHMARKING AND EVIDENCE BASED NATIONAL CLINICAL GUIDELINES FOR HEART FAILURE MANAGEMENT PROGRAMS: THE BENCH STUDY

Funding Source: National Heart Foundation of Australia Research Grants-in-Aid

This funding scheme (with a limit of $AU120,000 over two years) has the following underlying objectives in respect to providing research support:

- **Fund outstanding research across the areas of basic, clinical and public health.**
- Support the training of outstanding young cardiovascular researchers. across the areas of basic, clinical and public health research.
- Advocate for increased funding for cardiovascular research.

- Establish and maintain partnerships and alliances to support the generation, dissemination, use and funding support of cardiovascular research.
- Market Heart Foundation supported research outcomes and policy to external stakeholders.
- Communicate research activities and outcomes within the Heart Foundation.
- Support the translation and use of knowledge generated by cardiovascular research.

http://www.heartfoundation.com.au/index.cfm?page=198 (Accessed September 2006)

PROJECT SYNOPSIS

Chronic heart failure (CHF) a disabling, deadly and costly syndrome, is a major health issue deserving of a national health response. In the year 2000, it was estimated that >300,000 Australians were affected by CHF and required more than 100,000 acute hospitalizations. Despite the availability of effective treatments and management strategies, many patients with CHF receive suboptimal care. It is within this context that specialist CHF management programs have been developed. These programs have proven to be cost-effective in minimising the burden of CHF through improved management and applying best treatments, thereby reducing recurrent hospitalizations and prolonging survival. Unfortunately, there is considerable diversity in the intensity and range of strategies used to optimize the post-discharge management of CHF in Australia. Recent studies have highlighted the fact that not all approaches to CHF management result in the best outcomes for patients.

(i) The overall aim of this research project is to achieve the best possible outcomes for patients with CHF by developing a set of national benchmarks for the application and monitoring of CHF management programs in Australia. This will be achieved via a 3-stage process that will convene an international panel of experts to develop initial benchmarks, a clinical audit of Australian CHF programs and the development of Australian benchmarks to ensure quality care in the future.

INVESTIGATORS

Responsible Investigator:	Ms Andrea Driscoll (Early Career – PhD Candidate)
Senior Investigators:	Professor Simon Stewart (PhD Supervisor)
	Professor Andrew Tonkin (Highly credentialed Cardiologist)
	Dr Linda Worrall-Carter (PhD Supervisor)
Other Investigators:	Dr David Hare
	Dr Barbara Riegel
	Dr Patricia Davidson

STUDY AIMS

The overall aim of this research project is to develop national benchmarks and evidence-based clinical guidelines for heart failure management programs (HFMP) via a clinical audit of the characteristics and outcomes associated with every HFMP operating in Australia during the year 2005.

STUDY HYPOTHESES

Prior to the clinical audit a panel of international experts in HF management will designate the key characteristics and qualities of a cost-effective HFMP. Based on this information, we will test a number of specific hypotheses including:

1. Each HFMP is based on a cost-effective model of care suited to the local environment.
2. The core components of HF management in each HFMP are the same.
3. Each HFMP applies gold-standard pharmacologic and non-pharmacologic guidelines.
4. Patient outcomes (e.g. quality of life scores, morbidity and mortality rates) are equivalent for each HFMP (i.e. there is no relationship between quality of care and outcomes).

Based on a comparison between the proposed benchmarks for a cost-effective HFMP and the results of the clinical audit, a local panel of experts will determine minimum standards for the application and auditing of HFMP's in Australia to ensuring quality of care in HF.

SIGNIFICANCE

Chronic Heart Failure (CHF) is a major public health problem affecting >300,000 Australians and contributing to >1 million bed days/annum. Meta-analyses have shown that Heart Failure Management Programs (HFMP) are cost effective and improve patient outcomes. However, given the lack of national guidelines there is inherent variability in the types of HFMP's applied nationally. This study will use data from recent meta-analyses and panel of international experts to determine core components of a cost-effective HFMP. A clinical audit of HFMP's in Australia will identify the key characteristics of these relative to that designated by the expert panel. It will also compare key patient outcomes. Data from the clinical audit and recommendations from the expert panel will be reviewed by the research team to create Australian standards to ensure that the >60,000 patients/annum receive optimal care and benefit via improved outcomes.

STUDY BACKGROUND

As in most other developed countries, Australia is in the midst of an 'epidemic' of CHF. Associated with debilitating symptoms[1], a persistently high mortality rate[2,3,SS21], and frequent rehospitalisations[2] the population prevalence of this truly 'malignant' syndrome is likely to rise by 20–30% over the next 20 years[SS6]. Unfortunately, the public health response to CHF in Australia has been sub-optimal in comparison to other developed countries affected. This is both true in respect to both quantifying the burden it imposes on the population and the health care system and providing a coordinated and cost-effective response to the challenges and issues this contemporary epidemic engenders.

An 'epidemic' of chronic heart failure (CHF) in Australia. Although the epidemiologic profile of CHF in Australia is generally limited, there have been some attempts to address this important knowledge deficit. The CASE (Cardiac Awareness and Evaluation) Study (in which Professor Tonkin [SI–2] was an investigator) surveyed 341 GPs that were interested in CHF. The study found that of the 23,845 patient cohort, 2905 patients were diagnosed with CHF (13.2%).[AT10] Based upon these findings it was estimated that 300,000 Australians per annum were affected by this disease.[AT10] It is interesting to note that this prevalence was higher than that reported in comparable studies in other developed countries.[4] More recently a team led by Professor Stewart used the best available epidemiologic data to estimate that in the year 2000, over half a million Australians (3% of total population) were affected by CHF with 325,000 symptomatic patients/annum.[SS2] Hospital admissions for CHF, in the year 2000, were estimated at 100,000 admissions with a length of hospital stay of more than 1.4 million days: a prevalence rate of 526 hospitalisations and 7,400 days per 100,000/annum.[SS2] CHF accounted for over 10% of all hospitalisations for cardiovascular disease in the year 2000.[2] Interestingly, there is a decline in hospital bed availability of an average of 0.7% per year.[5] The estimated overall health care costs for this debilitating disease in 2000 was more than $1 billion with hospital costs accounting for >70% of the health care expenditure.[6] Indeed, the costs associated with CHF exceed that of all types of cancer.[2]

Key Point: These statistics and estimates reinforce the need for an Australian-wide response to the burden imposed by CHF in Australia: particularly as it will continue to rise for the foreseeable future. Consistent with the UK, USA, and Europe, the National Institute of Clinical Studies in Australia has identified CHF as a national health priority and Cardiac Society of Australia and New Zealand has developed a specialist-working group, under the leadership of Prof Henry Krum and Prof Stewart [SI-1], to address key issues relating to CHF.

Evidence supporting heart failure management programs (HFMP). In response to persistent and unacceptably high morbidity and mortality in CHF coupled with difficulties in applying gold-standard therapies, there has been increasing interest in the role of HFMP's to address these key issues in optimizing the management of CHF and providing the best possible individual and population health outcomes. In recent years, a series of appropriately powered randomised studies have shown that predominantly nurse-led multidisciplinary management programs reduce recurrent hospital stay and improve quality of life in typically older patients with CHF. When comparing HFMPs with the optimisation of drug therapy alone, patient outcomes such as quality of life, mortality, and readmission rates are similar or reduced for patients in a structured HFMP.[7,8] The implementation of HFMPs into the health care system has been prolific as preliminary evidence suggested that programs reduce costs, hospital readmission rates and patient morbidity, improve quality of life, functional capacity, and survival for CHF patients.[9–12,SS28] Recent meta-analyses have confirmed the efficacy of HFMP's overall in this regard.[13,14,SS3] For example, a recent meta-analysis has shown that multidisciplinary management prevents a total of 160 events/1000 patient years of treatment whereas treatment with digoxin, beta-blockers or angiotensin converting enzyme inhibitors prevents 28–63 events/1000 patient years of treatment.[SS3] The figure below [Figure 7.2] summaries the results of key randomised controlled trials concerning the effect that specialist post-discharge HFMPs have had in comparison to standard care in relation to length of stay.[SS8]

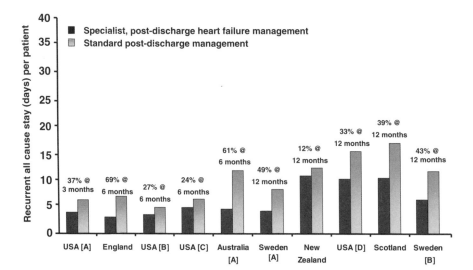

Figure 7.2. Impact of HFMP's on recurrent hospital stay relative to usual care

While the evidence to support HFMP's is strong, it is clear that some programs are likely to be superior than others in terms of cost-efficiency when tested under the same conditions (e.g. patient population and health care system). A recent panel of international experts who have led randomized studies of HFMP's and led by Professor Stewart [SI-1] and Barbara Riegel [OI–2] and including Professor's John McMurray[12], Mary Naylor[15] and Michael Rich[11] have suggested that HFMP's be categorized according to the following:

a. Mode of intervention: community-based versus specialist clinic versus remote access (i.e. telephone)
b. Complexity: singular focus (e.g. promote self-care or education alone) versus multidisciplinary models of care
c. Intensity: single or brief interventions versus prolonged follow-up.

Using the same categories, a team led by Professor McMurray and Professor Stewart have shown, in a meta-analysis that HFMP's involving multidisciplinary management via community-based or specialist clinics are most effective in reducing readmissions (RR 0.82 [95% CI 0.72–0.93]) and prolonging survival (RR 0.80 [95% CI 0.66–0.98]).[SS3]

Key Point: HFMPs are now integral to the post-discharge management of CHF and have been implemented widely.

Variability of heart failure management programs (HFMP). A major problem with the variability of HFMPs is that it has not been possible to identify which specific component of the program results in an improvement in patient outcomes such as mortality, morbidity, quality of life, and functional capacity. For example, one study found that one home visit post-discharge comprising of patient education resulted in a reduction in readmission rates and length of readmission hospital stay.[16] Other studies have investigated the effectiveness of inpatient education with post-discharge follow-up education on readmission rates and the length of readmission hospital stay and have found a reduction in both outcomes.[11,17,18]

Interestingly however, an independent relationship between discharge education and a reduction in readmission rates has not been found.[19,20] This variation in the approach to heart failure education between programs raises questions concerning evidence-based practice and the effectiveness of education in HFMPs. The role of education is one example, the literature also reveals gaps of evidence concerning: frequency and types of visits post-discharge, the type of HFMP (inpatient, outpatient, or outreach models), team members in the HFMP, medically-led or nurse-led coordination of care, NYHA classification of patients treated in the program, telephone follow-up, 24 hour telephone access, and point of discharge from the program and their effectiveness in improving patient outcomes.

In relation to models of HFMPs, meta-analysis has confirmed the effectiveness of specialised multidisciplinary heart failure programs on hospital readmission rates, mortality and cost-effectiveness.[13,14,SS3] However, there was inadequate data to determine the benefits of specific components within each program on patient outcomes.[13] There has been no evaluation of the relative benefits of nurse-led versus medically led coordination of care in HFMPs. There is little evidence for example, that a comprehensive multidisciplinary outreach HFMP incorporating several home visits and long term follow-up is any more effective in improving patient outcomes such as morbidity, quality of life, functional capacity, hospital readmission rates and survival, than a simple clinic based HFMP coordinated by a specialist nurse and cardiologist with one home visit. This makes funding of programs difficult especially within the context of fiscal restraints.

PILOT DATA

A preliminary study of post-discharge HFMPs within Australia was conducted by Professor Stewart (SI-01) to determine a baseline number and variability (unpublished data) Thirty-nine post-discharge HFMPs were identified from a systematic search of the Australian health care system in 2002 and sent a comprehensive 19-item questionnaire. The questionnaire specifically examined the characteristics including the model of care applied (e.g. home versus clinic-based), role of health care professionals and program funding.

All 39 HFMPs responded with six institutions (15%) indicating that their HFMPs had ceased operations due to a lack of funding. The comprehensive survey revealed a disproportion distribution of 33 active HFMPs operating throughout Australia: Vic and NSW each had 13 HFMPs, SA and WA 2 programs each and QLD three HFMPs at that time. In 2003 there were no HFMPs in the ACT, Tasmania, and Northern Territory. Overall, 4450 post-discharge CHF patients (median: 74; IQR: 24–147) were managed via HFMPs with 21% of programs managing >200 CHF patients/annum. As there are an estimated 40,000 CHF patients/annum who are discharged alive from metropolitan institutions throughout Australia, this represents only 11% of the potential caseload for an Australia-wide network of HFMPs.[10] Heterogeneity of HFMPs also exists in respect to: the model of care on which the HFMP is applied (70% applied a home-based program and 18% a specialist heart failure clinic), and program interventions (follow-up with a heart failure specialist and/or nurse occurred in 58% and 67% of cases, respectively, 51% of programs prevented nurses administering/titrating medications and discharge criteria existed in 52% of HFMPs with 29% having death as their criteria). Sustained funding was available to only 55% of these active HFMPs. Of these, funding was mainly provided by the institution itself (71%) or via research/ pharmaceutical company support (24%). The remaining programs (45%) did not have ongoing funding and their future was uncertain. Heterogeneity between HFMPs is prolific. Improving equity of access through developing benchmarks that are based upon quality cost-effective evidence is the foundation for evidence-based HFMPs.

Benchmarking of heart failure management programs (HFMP). Given the inherent variability of these programs (they have many components) and the expertise required to successfully manage CHF, it is of concern that there are no international or nationally-derived 'benchmarks' for evaluating pre-existing or future programs of this type. It is imperative to develop a general data set against which a service can evaluate its performance, quality and overall cost-effectiveness in order to maintain excellence and optimise patient outcomes. The proposed research will support the development of evidence-based national benchmarks and clinical guidelines for HFMPs. The development of benchmarks would begin to address the gaps in research through the identification of a national data set against which HFMPs can compare their outcomes to determine their quality and cost effectiveness. Benchmarking is a very powerful technique in driving best practice-orientated continuous improvement through programs and can be used as a tool to guide decision making for future HFMPs. The development of a benchmark will promote excellence in health care delivery. The strength of this research program is there are currently no national benchmarks for Australian HFMPs and there is a gap in the evidence concerning the effectiveness of specific interventions on patient outcomes.

RESEARCH PLAN

Overall Aim: The overall aim of this research project is to develop national benchmarks and evidence based clinical guidelines for HFMPs. This project involves a clinical audit of the characteristics and outcomes associated with every HFMP operating in Australia during the year 2005 (estimated total of 40 distinct programs).

Hypotheses: The following null hypotheses will be tested:

1. Relative to the guidelines developed by an international panel of experts, there will be no difference between HFMP's on the basis of the following:
   - Application of a cost-effective model of care suited to the local environment.
   - Core components of CHF management (e.g. each HFMP applies gold-standard pharmacologic and non-pharmacologic guidelines).
   - Patient outcomes (e.g. quality of life scores, morbidity and mortality rates).
2. If variances in the application of HFMP's and health outcomes do exist, there is no relationship between the quality of CHF care/management and health outcomes.

Part A: Identification of key components of cost-effective HFMP's

There has been an increasing focus on the implementation of HFMP's however there has been debate as to how best they can be applied and what the key components of CHF management are essential to achieving optimal outcomes. It is clear that there has been a clear need to establish expert consensus guidelines to both categorise HFMP's and recommend minimum standards for their application beyond those briefly mentioned in CHF guidelines. It is within this context that an international panel (involving Assoc. Prof. Davidson [OI–3] and facilitated by RI–1) is being co-led by Professor Simon Stewart and Assoc Professor Barbara Riegel during the *latter part of 2004* using an expert Delphi approach (via e-mail with follow-up at the ESC and AHA meetings) to develop these guidelines. Importantly, both Professor Simon Stewart and Assoc Professor Barbara Riegel have published key books on HFMP's from a European/NZ/Australian and USA perspective, respectively and have been involved in the practical implementation of such programs in Australia, UK and USA. Once these guidelines have been developed (expected early 2005), the research team will synthesize these into a list of key criteria by which HFMP's will be assessed using the information gathered as part of the systematic clinical audit.

Part B: Clinical audit of all Heart Failure Management Programs (HFMP)

The clinical audit will consist of two stages (see Figure 1 [Figure 7.3]). Stage I will involve auditing the aims, objectives, organizational characteristics and applied interventional strategies of each distinct HFMP in Australia (minimum of 40 HFMP's). Stage II will involve 6 month follow-up of 80 consecutive patients enrolled into at least 30 (75%) of these HFMP's to determine subsequent morbidity and mortality (overall n = 2,400 patients) with specific quality of life and functional data collected from 25 randomly selected patients from each program at baseline and 6 months (n = 750).

Stage 1: Auditing of HFMPs. Using the findings of the preliminary survey (unpublished data), a systematic review of the literature, review of meta-analyses, gold standard of non-pharmacological CHF management guidelines[21,22] and the international guidelines (developed from part A) a clinical audit tool using a modified version of the pilot study survey instrument (32 items) has been developed to identify variability in HFMPs. **Method:** prospective, cross-sectional survey design. **Sample:** a systematic search of the Australian health care system will be undertaken late 2004 to identify all HFMPs within Australia (at least 40 HFMPs are expected to be operational at this time).

Data collection: The following data will be collected from the HFMP co-coordinator:

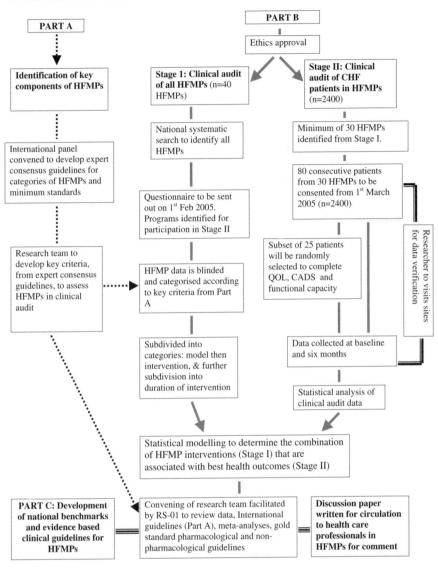

Figure 7.3. Research plan

- *HFMP profile:* size of hospital and program, hospital catchment area, NYHA class of patients, age of patients, mode of referral, admission and discharge criteria, and program aims and objectives
- *Infrastructure for program:* location and funding,
- *Staffing of HFMP:* members of the HFMP team, qualifications, role and specific duties, professional development, role of palliative care, frequency of team meetings,

- *HFMP model:* Model used such as inpatient, outpatient, or outreach model and duration of program. If a combination of models is used, what specific interventions comprise the combination.
- *Interventions of HFMP:* frequency and intensity of all interventions, reason for intervention, liaising with GP and community services, use of gold-standard pharmacotherapy (beta-blockers, ACE inhibitors, angiotensin II receptor antagonists, antiarrhythmics, cardiac glycosides, anticoagulants, vasodilators and aldosterone receptor antagonists), use of gold-standard non-pharmacological therapy (self care management strategies, patient compliance with treatment plan, patient and carer education, increased access and follow-up with Cardiologist and/or nurse specialist, telephone follow-up, exercise program, and co-ordination of care.
- *Program evaluation:* types of evaluation and frequency, other data collected to evaluate program, research conducted within the program, dissemination of evaluation results

HFMP Categorization: Based on the above, each program will be evaluated * to determine the presence/absence of the key components of HFMPs identified by the international panel in addition to any other features not prospectively listed but also applied by more than one HFMP. All programs will be allocated to one of three major categories (based on consensus, expert guidelines recently developed by Prof Stewart, Assoc Prof Riegel, Assoc Prof Naylor, Prof Rich and Prof. McMurray): Specialist heart failure clinic, Community-based management and Remote (e.g. telephonic support) management. Programs will be further delineated on the basis of singular versus multidimensional/multidisciplinary intervention and intensity of that intervention (i.e. brief versus sustained).

* HFMPs will be categorized independently and by a panel working with de-identified data in order to blind the process (RI-01, SI-01, SI-02, SI-03, OI-01, OI-03) prior to collation of patient follow-up data.

Study period: All HFMP Coordinators will be contacted by phone to discuss participation in the HFMP clinical audit and Stage II clinical audit of CHF patients, prior to sending an electronic survey on 1st February 2005 to be completed by 1st March 2005.

Stage II: Clinical audit of CHF patients: **Method:** prospective cross-sectional survey design. **Patient cohort and eligibility criteria:** patients with a diagnosis of CHF and who have had at least one hospital admission with CHF and/or CHF related discharge diagnosis. All of the patients must be enrolled in a post-discharge HFMP within Australia. **Patient recruitment:** At least 30 HFMPs willing to participate in the clinical audit of CHF patients were identified in Stage 1. All HFMPs will be sent a survey, clinical audit information sheet and patient consent form. The program coordinator in every HFMP will provide 80 consecutive patients, starting on the 1st of March 2005, with an information sheet prior to signing the consent form. A total of 2400 patients will be recruited from at least 30 HFMPs from March to September 2005.

Sample size: Stage II (patient follow-up) of this study has been powered to test the null hypothesis that there is no difference between each HFMP in respect to the composite primary endpoint of event-free survival (unplanned readmission or all-cause death) at 6 months. As such, a minimum of 80 subjects will have 80% power to detect a significant variance of 20% ($P < 0.05$) in the assumed event-free survival rate at 6 months of 50% between each HFMP. Most importantly, with a pooled analysis of 2400 patients and adjustment for the key components of intervention applied in addition to the broad category of program used to implement the key components of intervention (see below), this study will be sufficiently powered to detect a minimum 10% variation in specific morbidity and mortality rates between all 30 HFMP's subject to patient follow-up. Similarly, whilst there will be only specific quality of life and functional data for 25 randomly selected individuals from each HFMP, the total number of patients in whom these type of data will be collected will 750.

Baseline data collection: The following data will be collected from patients' medical records, and interviews of each patient with HFMP coordinator:

- Demographic data: *age, gender, ethnicity, education qualifications, marital status, social support, type of residence, rural or metropolitan area, cause and duration of CHF and medicare number.*
- Carlson's Co-morbidity scale
- *Functional capacity:* six minute walk test and ejection fraction (if available)
- *Medications:* type and dosage of medications (beta-blockers, ACE inhibitors, angiotensin II receptor antagonists, antiarrhythmics, cardiac glycosides, and aldosterone receptor antagonists).
- *Self care strategies*: daily weigh, strategies to manage weight diet, and fluid restriction.
- *#Quality of life:* Minnesota living with heart failure at 3 months
- *#Emotional well-being:* Cardiac Depression Scale (CADS)[23]
- *Knowledge about heart failure and disease implications*
- *Utilisation data:* Use of hospital services (Emergency department visits and hospital admissions) will be monitored via the patient's Medicare number and Hospital Insurance Commission.

*Data collected at baseline and six months. #Quality of life questionnaire and Cardiac Depression scale: a random sample of 25 patients/HFMP will be

contacted by phone and asked to complete the questionnaires at baseline and
six months

Study follow-up: The researcher will travel to all HFMPs throughout Australia
between 1st March 2005 and 1st March 2006 to audit and verify data collected.
All patients will be followed up for a minimum of 6 months. Data collection
will occur at baseline and 6 months. **Major end-points:** The primary end-point
will be event-free survival from all-cause mortality and unplanned readmission
at 6 months. Secondary end-points will be all-cause hospital stay, CHF-related
hospital readmission and stay (calculated as the number of days of unplanned
hospital readmission/number of follow-up days). Other data that will be examined are changes in quality of life (QOL), functional capacity, and emotional
well being. **Statistical analysis of Stage II:** Time-dependent morbidity and
mortality data from the follow-up of all 2400 patients will be used to construct
event-free survival, all-cause mortality and accumulative readmission curves
for each category of HFMP (e.g. low-intensity, multidisciplinary community-
based management versus high-intensity, multidisciplinary, specialist heart
failure clinic). For dichotomous outcomes (e.g. event-free survival), step-wise
multiple logistic regression models with entry of baseline clinical and demographic patient characteristics, prescribed pharmacologic therapy, key components of intervention and overall category of the HFMP the patient has
been exposed to will be used to determine significant correlates of 6-month
morbidity and mortality. Further modeling will be undertaken to determine
which combination of interventions, when adjusting for potential baseline
confounders is associated with the best health outcomes. Emergency department and inpatient hospital activity will be monitored based on coding of
admissions using the WHO International Classification of Disease system and
the HIC, using the patient's Medicare number. Multiple analysis of variance
will be used to compare health care utilization rates (e.g. all-cause hospital
stay/patient/month of follow-up), cardiac depression score and QOL score to
determine independent predictors of outcome.

Part C: Development of benchmarks and evidence based clinical guidelines for HFMPs

The research team who are experts in CHF management, facilitated by RI–01,
will meet to advise and guide the process for developing national benchmarks
and evidence based clinical practice guidelines for Australian HFMPs. These
will be developed in conjunction with the International guidelines (developed
in Part A), synthesis of meta-analyses, available data from this project, gold
standard pharmacologic[AT12] and non-pharmacologic guidelines[21,22]. A discussion paper concerning the national benchmarks and guidelines will be written
and circulated to health professionals involved in HFMPs for comments. This
will ensure that the benchmarks and guidelines are relevant to clinical practice

and is also consistent with internal validity of the method and data analysis that are used to develop the benchmarks and guidelines.

REFERENCES

1. Juenger J, *et al.* Health-related quality of life in patients with congestive heart failure: Comparison with other chronic diseases & relation to functional variables. *Heart* 2002; 87: 235–41.
2. AIHW. 2001. *Heart, stroke and vascular disease:Australian Facts 2001.* Perth, Australian Institute Health and Welfare, the National Heart Foundation, and National stroke Foundation of Australia.
3. Levy D, *et al.* Long-term trends in the incidence of and survival with heart failure. *N Engl J Med* 2002; 347: 1397–1402.
4. Mair FS, *et al.* Prevalence, aetiology and management of heart failure in general practice. *Br J General Practice* 1996; 46: 77–79.
5. AIHW. *Australian Hospital Statistics 2001–2002.* Canberra: AIHW. 2003.
6. AIHW: Jamrozik K, *et al. Monitoring the incidence of cardiovascular disease in Australia.* Cardiovascular Disease Series No. 17. AIHW Cat. No. CVD 16. Canberra: AIHW. 2001.
7. Hjalmarson A, *et al.* Effects of controlled-release metoprolol on total mortality, hospitalisations, and well-being in patients with heartfailure: the Metoprolol CR/XL Randomised Intervention Trial in Congestive Heart Failure (MERIT-HF). MERIT-HF Study Group. *JAMA.* 2000; 283: 1295– 1302.
8. The Cardiac Insufficiency Bisoprolol Study II (CIBIS-II): a randomised trial. *Lancet.*1999; 353: 9–13.
9. Kasper, E. K., *et al.* A randomised trial of the efficacy of multidisciplinary care in heart failure outpatients at high risk of hospital readmission. *J Am Coll Cardiol.* 2002; 39: 471–480.
10. Krumholz, H. M., *et al.* Randomised trial of an education and support intervention to prevent readmission of patients with heart failure. *J Am Coll Cardiol.* 2002; (39): 83–89.
11. Rich, M. W., *et al.* A Multidisciplinary intervention to prevent the readmission of elderly patients with congestive heart failure. *New England J of Med.* 1995; 333: 1190–1195.
12. Blue, L., E. Lang, *et al.* (2001). 'Randomised controlled trial of specialist nurse intervention in heart failure.' *BMJ* 323(7315): 715–8.
13. Mc Alister, F. A. *et al.* A systematic review of randomized trials of disease management programs in heart failure. *Am J of Med* 2001; 110: 378–384.
14. Phillips, C.O., *et al.* (2004). 'Comprehensive Discharge Planning with Postdischarge Support for Older Patients with Congestive Heart Failure: A Meta-analysis' *JAMA:* 291(11): 1358–1367.
15. Naylor, M. D. and K. M. McCauley (1999). 'The effects of a discharge planning and home follow-up intervention on elders hospitalized with common medical and surgical cardiac conditions.' *J Cardiovasc Nurs* 14(1): 44–54.
16. Holst, D. P. *et al.* Improved outcomes from a comprehensive management system for heart failure. *European Journal of Heart Failure.* 2001; (3): 619–625.

17. Cline, C. M. *et al.* Cost effective management programme for Heart Failure reduces hospitalisation. *Heart.* 1988; (80): 442–446.
18. Weinberger, M., Smith DM, Katz BP, & Moore PS. The cost-effectiveness of intensive postdischarge care. *Med Care.* 1988; 11: 1092–1101.
19. Jaarsma, T. *et al.* Effects of education and support on self-care and resource utilisation in patients with heart failure. *European Heart Journal.* 1999; (20): 673–682.
20. Weinberger, M. *et al.* Does increased access to primary care reduce hospital readmissions *N Engl J Med.* 1996; 334: 1441–1447. Doughty, R. N. et al. *European Heart Journal* 2002; 23: 139–146.
21. McKay I & Stewart S. Optimising the day-to-day management of patients with chronic heart failure. In *Specialist Nurse Intervention in Chronic Heart Failure: From research to practice.* S Stewart & L Blue (Editors) BMJ Books, London. 2004.
22. Moser DK, *et al.* Non-pharmacologic management of heart failure. In *Caring for the heart failure patient.* S Stewart, DK Moser & DR Thompson (Editors). Martin Dunitz, London, UK. 2004.
23. Hare, D Davis, C. Cardiac Depression Scale: Validation of a new depression scale for cardiac patients. *Journal of Psychosomatic research.* 1996; 40(4): 379–386.

BUDGET

A total of $AU 24,000 was requested to support Ms Driscoll's activities given that she was already a recipient of a Heart Foundation Postgraduate Research Fellowship.

APPLICATION 2: CARDIAC-ARIA: MEASURING THE ACCESSIBILITY TO CARDIOVASCULAR SERVICES IN RURAL REMOTE AUSTRALIA VIA APPLIED GEOGRAPHICAL SPATIAL TECHNOLOGY (GIS)

Funding Source: The Australian Research Council Linkage Program

This funding program is under the umbrella of the National Competitive Grants Program. Under Backing Australia's Ability, the Australian Government's 2001 innovation action plan, increased funding supports research in Linkage programs. The underlying objectives of the scheme are as follows:

• To encourage excellent collaborative research within universities and across the innovation system
• To contribute to a strong knowledge economy
• To create opportunities for cooperation with related programmes across Commonwealth portfolios
• To facilitate international linkages both within universities and industry
• To encourage industry oriented research training.

http://www.arc.gov.au/grant_programs/linkage.htm   (Accessed   September 2006)

STUDY AIMS

The specific aims of the study are to;

1. Map the type and location of cardiovascular services currently available in Australia, relative to the distribution of individuals who currently have symptomatic cardiovascular disease (CVD);
2. Determine, by expert panel, what are the minimal requirements for comprehensive cardiovascular health support in a metropolitan and rural community and
3. Derive a ranking or weighting classification (based on the ARIA Model) for each of Australia's 11,338 rural and remote population centres according to their level of access to the minimal requirements for comprehensive cardiovascular health support in a community.

BACKGROUND

Cardiovascular disease (CVD) is one Australia's most important public health issues.[1] In a cardiovascular emergency (heart attack or stoke) every minute counts, for the prevention of CVD every healthy year counts. In 2001, there were 50,294 deaths and 3.67 million people affected by CVD.[2] Of the 10 National health priority areas, the disease burden associated with CVD (22%) exceeds that of any other disease group.[3] Despite a reduction in mortality over the last few decades, nearly 4 in 10 (16.4%) Australians die from CVD each year.[4,5] With increases in life expectancy and an ageing population it is expected that 25 % of Australians will have CVD by 2051. Similar trends are occurring in most industrialised countries.[1] Furthermore, CVD contributes to significant morbidity and impaired quality of life.[1]

It is within this context that more than one million Australians suffer from long-term illness and disability, from conditions associated with CVD. There is also evidence to suggest that poor CVD outcomes are not equally shared across the entire population. Higher prevalence rates of CVD are evident for males, lower socioeconomic groups and some geographical locations – particularly rural and remote areas.[3] CVD is one of the most costly chronic diseases.[3] In Australia the total health care cost of CVD was $5.5 billion between 2001 and 2002, and nearly two thirds was spent on people aged 65 years and older.[5] Hospital services contributed to nearly half of this expenditure, followed by pharmaceuticals (26%), medical services provided out of hospital (14%) and aged care. Over the past decade (1994–2004) inflation-adjusted expenditure for cardiovascular disease has increased by 28%.[1] Given the ageing of Australia's population[6], a sustained capacity to deliver appropriate health care will pose a significant challenge for future governments.

There is a strong relationship between CVD and a range of risk factors and health related conditions.[7] Evidence suggests that modifying or eliminating these would have long-term benefits, in reducing the future burden of CVD. However an individual's risk of illness cannot be considered in isolation from the population to which he or she belongs.[8] Therefore, there is a need to better understand the relationship between populations at risk, social and environmental forces and demographic changes. Accurate information is also required in respect to those factors likely to influence our ability to meet the needs of Australians who are already living with CVD in addition to those who will make the transition to symptomatic CVD in the near future, for example obese children. (Fig 1) Moreover, given the size of the CVD epidemic, it is imperative we generate future models that determine where we are likely to succeed, or fail in our current endeavours to positively influence the preventative measures and services available to the Australian population.

CARDIAC-ARIA: development of a public heath tool to map the current services available for management and prevention of CVD in Australia

Projecting population-based figures to describe any particular health care condition, without taking account of the unique geography and social fabric of Australia is, of <u>limited value</u> for 'informed' future planning. It is within this context that the study team has already <u>collaborated</u> to undertake research utilising geographical information system (GIS) technology to identify the spatial distribution of chronic heart failure in relation to specialist and general practitioner services in Australia (Fig 2) [Figure 7.4]. This work will inform the development of a national Australian geographical cardiac index, using methodologies similar to those used for the Accessibility and Remoteness Index of Australia (ARIA),[9] (Fig 3) GP-ARIA and Ph-ARIA.[10]

SIGNIFICANCE AND INNOVATION

A unique feature of this study will be our use of 'state of the art' GIS modelling technology, to map the spatial distribution of CVD in relation to current

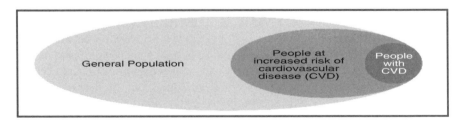

Figure 7.4. Diagram of population at risk of cardiovascular disease: NHF of Australia, Focus for Core Activities (2005)

cardiovascular health care services, while varying the effects of differing population risk profiles, socio-demographic characteristics and demographic change associated with progressive ageing.

GIS technology has been used extensively to map the spatial–temporal distribution of infectious diseases and to identify 'hotspots'/clusters of disease activity. Recently GIS have been recognized as a valuable tool to assist in health services planning, but its undoubted potential to for utilization in healthcare is under valued.

There is clear evidence to suggest that inequities in health outcomes exist between socio-economically advantaged and disadvantaged groups,[1] the gap is widening and poor CVD outcomes are not equally shared across the entire population. People from socio-economically disadvantaged groups have a poorer risk profile and are more likely to die from CVD than those from more privileged backgrounds. One of the most disadvantaged groups in Australia are Aboriginal and Torres Strait Islander people who experience a 2.6 fold increase in CVD mortality and a 1.4 higher rate of hospitalization, compared to other Australians. Forty-one per cent of all CVD deaths and 30% of Indigenous deaths occur in rural and remote areas of Australia.[12]

Together with significant health inequalities, inequalities also exist in access to and delivery of health care services in Australia.[13] This is particularly evident for specialist cardiac services in rural and remote areas, where few Cardiologists live and work, and a large proportion of the burden of health care falls upon the local GP, whose numbers have diminished in recent times.[14] With the trend to down-grade local rural hospitals to aged care centres, or close them completely, there is an increasing need for people with CVD to travel, often long distances, to larger urban or city-based cardiac care specialist centres to receive appropriate and timely care.[15] Given that people with CVD take more health actions than the average Australian [5,6] the added financial costs associated with travel imposes a significant burden on our older population.

It is well known that the prevalence of CVD in Australia will rise with the progressive ageing of its population: Australia has the 3rd highest population increase in people aged >65 years and is a world leader in population growth in those aged >85 years.[2] Moreover, Australian Bureau of Statistics population projection data indicates that there will be a shift in the age structure of Australians with the proportion of persons aged >65 years projected to increase from 14.5% in 2000 to 31.5% (+220,000 persons) in 2051. Conversely, the number of persons aged 0–64 years is predicted to decline from 1,280,922 to 971,306 persons.[16] Much of the expected increase in Australia's older population has been attributed to the impact of the ageing 'Baby Boomer' cohort, decreasing fertility rates and a drop in the proportion of young people.[17] Compared to previous generations, the current generation of older Australians is more educated and experience better health.[2] This enhanced status, particularly in regard to health, has been attributed to continuous improvements in medical techniques and treatments, improved diet, increased access to medical services, and generally improved life-styles.[17] The healthy ageing of Australia's older population has also resulted in significant retirement migration from metropolitan to non-metropolitan areas (in the 65 plus age group) and contributed to increased population growth, similar to that seen in major cities, and a blurring of the sharp boundaries once drawn around Australia's major cities. However, population growth in non-metropolitan areas is variable with more accessible geographical locations, such as the urban fringes and better watered areas, experiencing growth and more remote areas in decline.[18] Regrettably, services in these areas, including health services, have not kept pace with the changing face of Australia's non-metropolitan population. Some communities, situated in the fringes of major cities, for example, are located between 50 and 80 kilometres away from cardiac services. The lack of appropriate and timely healthcare in areas outside of major cities has serious implications for Australia's older people where the demand for health care services is more acute [see Figures 7.5 and 7.6].[15]

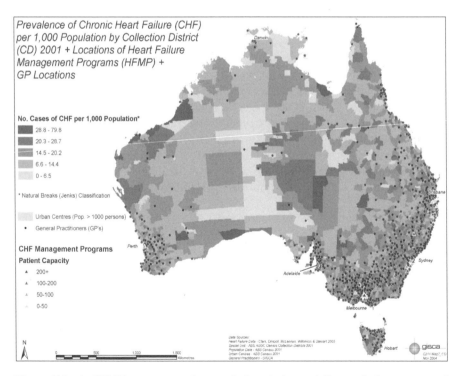

Figure 7.5. A GISCA map: prevalence of chronic heart failure relative to general practice and specialist chronic heart failure services

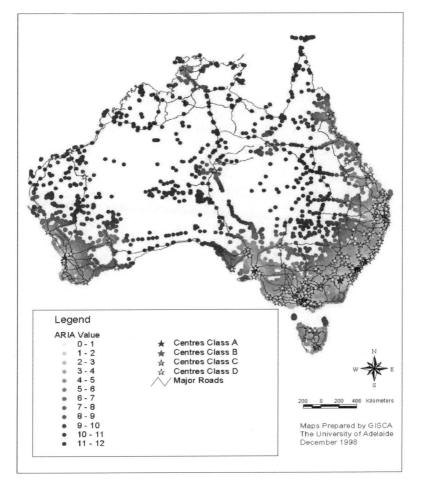

Figure 7.6. GISCA ARIA Project 1998: map of population localities, service centres and major road networks

APPROACH AND TRAINING

Conceptual framework

Maps have been used as a public health tool for over 150 years. A well-known example exists in early infectious disease epidemiology and John Snow's mapping of the cholera epidemics in London in 1854. More recently, geographical information system (GIS) technology and the increasing availability of health data, together with improvements in data collection techniques, has made it possible to develop a wide range of functions to enhance early mapping procedures. GIS is a digital computerised map (see Fig. 2 above) [Figure 7.5], with associated databases, that allows data from a variety of sources to be linked to places on a map using a process called *geo-coding*.

Design

This study will be a collaborative **4 stage geo-coding project** where CVD data obtained by systematic review, Delphi survey methods and implementation of previously modelled geo-codes (GP-ARIA and Ph-ARIA)

METHODS

The methods for **CARDIAC-ARIA** will be based on that used to develop the Accessibility and Remoteness Index of Australia (ARIA).[9] ARIA is a comparative measure of geographic remoteness for all populated localities (or aggregated areas) throughout Australia. ARIA determines geographic remoteness and accessibility in terms of the distance the population of each town or locality must travel to reach services. Populated localities are defined as any of over 11,000 populated centres in Australia. Service centres are the populated centres with a population of 1000 or more at the time of the 2001 census. The ARIA methodology has successfully been adapted for the development of a GP and Pharmacy accessibility index [10]. The **CARDIAC-ARIA** index will be developed for all towns in Australia. Similar to the ARIA index, it can then be aggregated to any other area unit such as a Local Government Area, Statistical Local Area, Postcode, Census Collection District or any other user defined catchments. This will allow the incorporation of population data for any of these areas to be included so that estimates of population at risk can be easily calculated. The development of **CARDIAC-ARIA** will involve several key stages [Figure 7.7]:

Stage 1   **Compilation of data on the type and location of cardiac services in Australia**: A systematic search of Australian health care system operational data (e.g. professional societies, AIHW, AHMAC Workforce data, state health departments and NICS) and existing data (maintained by GISCA) will be undertaken to identify the location and type of all cardiac services. These data will be systematically catalogued and prepared for **Stage 2** below.

Stage 2   **Classification of specialist cardiac services throughout Australia**: All towns (localities) in Australia that provide cardiac services will then be categorized on a scale ranging from 1 to 6 to delineate the extent of specialist care immediately available at that location: a score of 1 indicating the highest level of service provision while a score of 6 will indicate the complete absence of cardiac services. For example it is expected that Sydney and Melbourne would be categorized as a Level 1 service location because these cities have cardiac transplant services available within their city boundaries.

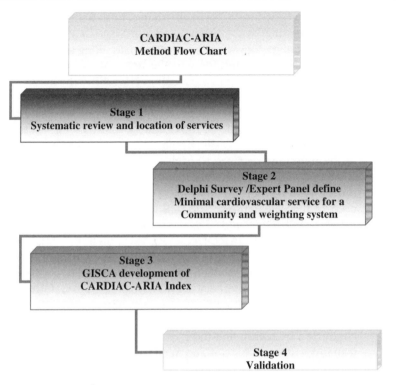

Figure 7.7. CARDIAC-ARIA method flow chart

Conversely, Adelaide and Hobart may not be categorized as providing Level 1 services, despite being capital cities, on the basis of the absence of cardiac transplant services. Using the same methodology used to create ARIA all locations with a classification Level of 1 to 5 will be designated as cardiac service centres and used for the calculation of CARIAC-ARIA. Importantly, the category allocation will be undertaken once all the data from *Stage 1* has been collected, and will initially be compiled internally by the expert research team. The team will then convene an external expert reference group (led by Prof Andrew Tonkin) who will independently review and validate the classification of services inherent to CARDIAC-ARIA. Once consensus agreement is reached by this expert panel, these data will be incorporated into the GIS database along with pre-existing data (e.g. location of GP and pharmacy services).

Stage 3 ***Computation of CARDIAC-ARIA***: Once the service centres are classified in *Stage 2*, the same methodology used to develop ARIA will be followed to compute CARDIAC-ARIA. Network analysis will be conducted on the entire Australian road network coverage. Distance measurements were generated from all populated localities (11,338 localities) to all urban centres with a cardiac service (centres classified as between 1 and 5 in Stage 2). All distances will be calculated by following the shortest path along the road network from the populated localities to the urban centres. The minimum distance from each populated location (11,338) to the nearest centre for each of the five levels, will be calculated. Statistics for the mean and standard deviation will be calculated for distances to each of the five levels. The ratio of the distances to the mean will be calculated for each of the 11,338 populated locations. The ratios for each of the minimum distance to each of the five levels will then added to form a single accessibility value for each populated location. A threshold maximum travel distance of three times the mean will be used in the calculations. This will give a continuous variable with values of between 0 and 15 as the measure of access to cardiac services. The values of CARDIAC-ARIA will then interpolated onto a one kilometre regular grid for the whole of Australia. From this regular grid, an average value for CARDIAC-ARIA will be calculated for each collection district unit, postcode area, statistical local area and local government area in Australia.

Stage 4   ***An initial validation of the CARDIAC-ARIA***: Ratings will be conducted by comparing the rankings to exiting data such as Australian Institute of Health and Welfare CVD mortality and rates.

PhD AND POST DOCTORAL SCHOLARSHIP

This project has scope for the scholarship of two Australian Postgraduate Award PhDs, one each in the fields of cardiovascular health and GIS and the early career research development of one or more post doctoral candidates under the supervision of the team of internationally renowned researchers, mentors and supervisors involved in this project.

PARTNER ORGANISATION COMMITMENT AND COLLABORATION

This project relies on the collaboration of 5 key partners

1. The University of South Australia (Administration and Cardiovascular research)
2. The University of Adelaide (GISCA)
3. The University of Queensland (Rural and Remote and Epidemiology)
4. Monash University /The National Heart Foundation (Prof Andrew Tonkin)
5. Alphapharm pharmaceuticals

Each partner brings its own team of international experts to combine to produce a world class tool not previously developed in any other country.

Industry Partner commitment

Alphapharm is Australia's leading supplier of prescription pharmaceuticals. While the company specializes in bringing patent-expired medicines to market, Alphapharm also researchers and developes innovative medicines to treat metabolic and cardiovascular diseases, and to prevent the development and spread of cancers.

Alphapharm has a strong focus on the prevention and treatment of cardiovascular disease (CVD) and sponsor education, information and research activities in the field of CVD. Our wide range of cardiovascular products and our strong commitment to encouraging the quality use of medicines complement this.

Alphapharm is therefore a strong supporter of the abovementioned project to map the current and future need for, and accessibility to, cardiovascular services in Australia via applied geographical spatial technology (GISCA). Apart from Alphapharm's strong and ongoing commitment generally to supporting research, they are especially interested in initiatives that will help to increase cardiovascular health and reduce the burden of cardiovascular disease. In particular, Alphapharm will benefit from supporting the GISCA/ CARDIAC-ARIA project, as the results will assist in strategic planning around sales and marketing issues for the company. The results will enable Alphapharm to target particular population localities, which could be a focus for future company-facilitated educational programs.

Alphapharm welcome the opportunity to be involved in a prestigious and internationally recognized collaborating team made up of five organizations, including three universities and two industry partners. The chief investigators – Professors Simon Stewart (University of South Australia), Andrew Tonkin (National Heart Foundation), Graeme Hugo (GISCA University of Adelaide) and David Wilkinson (University of Queensland) form an impressive list of leading researchers in their fields of expertise.

Alphapharm and the University research teams, already have a track record of collaboration in the areas of education and sponsorship. For example, Alphapharm have recently supported the development of collaborative research and educational networks for involving specialist cardiac nurses. This project will extend these alliances, to the research level and pending successful outcomes will provide opportunity to further extended research collaboration.

NATIONAL BENEFIT

This unique and innovative project has the potential to deliver a powerful tool to both highlight and combat the burden of CVD in Australia with:

- The ability to identify geographical 'hotspots' where there is likely to be a mismatch between demand for and actual provision of cardiovascular services.

- The development of **CARDIAC-ARIA** will inform future research that aims to determine if the prevalence of CVD is associated with accessibility and remoteness to cardiac services.
- The capability to update established models as validated Australian CVD burden and risk factor data emerges: all of this data can then be made freely accessible through the World Wide Web.

Overall, this research has the potential to greatly facilitate the ARC Research Priority 2:

Promoting and Maintaining good health and well being for all Australians; Ageing well, ageing productively; and strengthening Australia's social and economic fabric, by ensuring an equitable distribution of quality services to Australian currently living with CVD and therefore optimising health outcomes.

COMMUNICATION OF RESULTS

As this project will be part of two APAI PhDs, all aspects of the project will be published as part of the requirements of scholarship in relevant peer viewed journals. The track record of all CI's clearly indicates a track record of commitment to publication and dissemination of research in addition to translation into the real-world.

STUDY TIMELINES

Project Stages	Year 1 2007	Year 2 2008	Year 3 2009	Comments
Ethics and/or Institutional approval Enrolment of APAIs Strategic meeting of CIs	➡			Complete March 2007
Stage One Systematic review of CVD services				Complete and publish December 2007
Stage Two Delphi Survey/Expert	➡			Complete Stage 2 June 2008

Panel define Minimal cardiovascular service for a Community and weighting system	➡			
Stage Three GISCA development of CARDIAC-ARIA Index		➡		Complete Stage3 December 2008
Stage Four Validation			➡	Complete June 2009
Completion of reports and publications Submission of APAI PhDs			➡	Project completion 2009

RESEARCH TEAM

	CI/PI	Role	Responsibility	Contribution
1	**Prof Simon Stewart**	CI	Supervision and overseeing the Cardiovascular data for geo-code developments	Cardiovascular health and research expert
2	**Prof Andrew Tonkin**	CI	Development of minimal services for community CVD support	Leadership of consultant with specialist cardiologists
3	**Prof David Wilkinson**	CI	Supervision and overseeing the Rural and remote health and epidemiological data for geo-code developments	Rural and remote Epidemiology expert

4	Robyn Clark	CI (Early Career Development)	Project management. Coordination of collaborators/team Supervision of APAI (CVD)	Rural and remote cardiovascular health and information communication technology expertise
5	Neil Coffee	CI (Early Career Development)	Coordination of GIS component GIS Training of APAI (GISCA)	GIS Expert
6	Kerena Eckert	CI (Early Career Development)	Development of cardiovascular epidemiology data Supervision of expertise APAI (CVD)	Rural and remote epidemiology and cardiovascular health
7	Peter Astles	PI (Industry Partner)	Partner in Industry consultant. Project steering committee member	External peer review
8	Marian Milligan	PI (Industry Partner)	Partner in Industry consultant. Project steering committee member	External peer review
9	APAI (PhD CVD)	Cardiovascular Health	Training in collection processing and publication of CVD data for geo-coding	PhD Research training and publication
10	APAI (PhD GISCA)	GIS	Training in GIS processing of geo-coding and publication of results	PhD Research training and publication

REFERENCES

1. Australian Institute of Health and Welfare (AIHW). *Heart, stroke and vascular diseases – Australian facts 2004. AIHW Cat No. CVD 27 http:www.aihw.gov.au/ publications/health/*. Canberra 2004.

2. Australian National Heart Foundation. *Cardiovascular disease: http://www. heartfoundation.com.au/downloads/cvd.htm* 2001.
3. Australian Institute of Health and Welfare (AIHW). Health System Costs of Cardiovascular Diseases and Diabetes in Australia 1993–1994 http://www. aihw.gov.au/publications/healthhsccdda93-4/hsccdda93-4.pdf. Health and Welfare Expenditure Series No.5.
4. Australian Institute of Health and Welfare. *Population ageing and the economy.* Canberra: AIHW; 1999.
5. National Heart Foundation of Australia. *The cost of cardiovascular disease in Australia.* Canberra: NHF; 2004.
6. Peterson C, Walker C, Southern D. From episodic treatment to chronic disease management: Shifting the over 65 population to an alternative model of care. Available from http://www.priory.com/fam/chrondisman.htm. Assessed Feb 25 2005.
7. O'Brien K. *Living dangerously: Australians with multiple risk factors for cardiovascular disease. Australia Institute of Health and Welfare, Bulletin 24 Cat No. AUS 57.* Canberra: AIHW; 2005.
8. Berkman L, Kawachi I. *Social Epidemiology.* New York: Oxford University Press, Inc.; 2000.
9. Commonwealth of Australia (2003). Measuring remoteness: Accessibility and Remoteness Index of Australia (ARIA) http://www.gisca.adelaide.edu.au/ products_services/aria2_about.html.
10. GISCA. *Pharmacy Access/Remoteness Index of Australia (PhARIA) http://www. gisca.adelaide.edu.au/projects/pharia.html* 2004.
11. Meltzer M, Cox N, Fukuda K. Modelling the economic impact of pandemic influenza in the United States: Implication for setting priorities for intervention. Available at: http://wwwcdc.gov/ncidod/eid/vol5no5/melt_back.htm. (Accessed Feb 25). 1999.
12. Australian Institute of Health and Welfare (AIHW). *Rural, regional and remote health: a study on mortality. AIHW cat. No. PHE 45. (Rural Health Series no.2).* Canberra 2003.
13. Australian Institute of Health and Welfare. *The Health and Welfare of Australia's Aboriginal and Torres Strait Island Peoples*: Australian Bureau of Statistics (ABS) Cat 4704.0; 2003.
14. Cameron I. Retaining a medical workforce in rural Australia. *MJA.* 1998; 169: 293–294.
15. Lyle D. Infrastructure support for rural practitioners. In: Wilkinson D, Blue I, Eds. *The New Rural Health.* Vol 1. South Melbourne: Oxford Press Pty Ltd; 2002: 260–272.
16. Australian Bureau of Statistics. Australian social trends 1999 Population – population projections: Our aging population. *http://wwwabs.gov.au/Ausstats/abs@nsf/.* 2004.
17. Strategic Planning & Research Branch. *The impact of ageing: A literature review*: Department of Human Services, Government of South Australia; August 2003.
18. Clark RA, McLennan S, Eckert K, Dawson A, Wilkinson D, Stewart S. Heart Failure beyond city limits. Rural and Remote Health Available from: http://rrh. deakin.edu.au. 2005; 5: 443.

BUDGET

The following budget was requested to primarily support two PhD scholarships and the cost of generating the geo-maps of Australia's cardiac services:

Column 1	2	3	4		5	6
Source of funds	ARC	University	Eligible Partner Organisations		Other	Total
			Cash	In-kind		
TOTAL DIRECT COSTS	158688	301779	39990	144990	0	645447

APPLICATION 3: WHICH HEART FAILURE INTERVENTION IS MOST COST-EFFECTIVE AND CONSUMER FRIENDLY IN REDUCING HOSPITAL CARE: THE WHICH TRIAL

Funding Source: The Australian Health and Medical Research Council's Health Service Research Program (Round 3 of funding)

This program supports multi-disciplinary research into how financing arrangements, organisational structures and processes, health technologies and social factors affect the quality, cost and availability of, and access to, health care. As part of the peer-review process, priority is afforded to research which:

• Addresses significant gaps in evidence required for Australia 's most important policy and practice issues;
• Covers issues related to the Australian Government's National Research Priorities or National Health Priority Areas and or Aboriginal and Torres Strait Islander health and access to health services;
• Has the potential to develop new productive partnerships between researchers, policy makers, health service providers and citizens.

In addition to the National Health Priority Areas and National Research Priorities, Round 3 encouraged applicants to research Aboriginal and Torres Strait Islander health and access to health services.

BACKGROUND: OPTIMISING OUTCOMES IN CHRONIC HEART FAILURE – A NATIONAL PRIORITY!

It is now well recognised that chronic heart failure (CHF), a costly [1], debilitating and deadly [2] clinical syndrome, has emerged as a major public health issue within Australia's ageing population.[3] Data from two notable

Australian studies of heart failure in primary care (the CASE Study [4]) and a more recent population study (the Canberra Heart Study [5]) are consistent with recent estimates of the burden imposed by CHF on Australia's health care system in the year 2000:

- Approximately 325,000 Australians (58% male) had typical symptoms of shortness of breath and fatigue associated with the syndrome of CHF.
- There were around 100,000 CHF-related hospitalisations involving 1.4 million days of hospital stay: a prevalence rate of 526 hospitalisations & 7,400 days per 100,000/annum.
- Of these hospital admissions, more than 80% were likely to involve patients aged >65 years: 89% of hospital stay attributable to this older and more fragile cohort of patients.
- The total cost of CHF to the Australian health care system was more than $1 billion.[6]

In the absence of an <u>absolute</u> cure for progressive ventricular dysfunction and the most common precursors of CHF (heart disease and hypertension), the number of older Australians affected by this syndrome is likely to increase by at least 20–30% within the next 20 years [6]; particularly if current rates of diabetes and obesity in middle-aged Australians persist. [7] Addressing the enormous and rising health status and health care problem engendered by CHF is, therefore, directly relevant to National Research (***Promoting & Maintaining Good Health: Ageing well, ageing productively***) and National Health Priorities (***Cardiovascular Health***).

The emergence of Chronic Heart Failure Management Programs

In response to the high burden associated with CHF, in particular hospital admissions, dedicated CHF management programs (CHF-MPs) have been developed to optimise health outcomes in a cost-effective way. These multi-disciplinary programs target recently hospitalised patients in an effort to opti-mise the ongoing /long-term management of CHF including post acute discharge care within the community. A series of recent meta-analyses have confirmed the benefits of CHF-MPs in reducing readmission rates, improving quality of life, reducing costs and prolonging survival. For example we have demonstrated that patients exposed to the intervention arms of these studies were significantly less likely to be readmitted (17% risk reduction) or die (16% risk reduction).[8] The following two major forms of CHF-MP are found to have the greatest impact on health outcomes in meta-analyses (25% reduced risk of unplanned hospitalisation):

- Multidisciplinary, specialist CHF clinic (**clinic-based intervention**)
- Multidisciplinary, community-based management (**home-based intervention**)

Applying Chronic Heart Failure Management Programs: Which one?

Consistent with the above data, CHF-MP's now form part of the gold-standard management of CHF in Australia with the highest level of evidence cited.[6] Also consistent with the *National Service Improvement Framework for Heart Stroke and Vascular Disease*, there has been increasing interest in implementing CHF-MP's throughout Australia. However, our NHF-funded BENCH Study has clearly demonstrated that funding for these programs has been inconsistent and, reflecting the fact that various models of care have been reported in the literature there is marked heterogeneity in applying the evidence. [9] At best, only 20% of Australian patients with CHF and living in metropolitan regions have access to CHF-MP's following an acute hospitalisation. Within this context, all recent meta-analyses of CHF-MP's have called for appropriately powered, head-to-head studies of clinic and home-based multidisciplinary intervention to ultimately decide which is most cost-effective in practice. Given other potential differences in the burden imposed by these programs on both the patient and their family/carer, [6, 10] there is an urgent need to determine which of the most effective forms of CHF-MP (home *vs.* clinic-based management) will serve the Australian population best in terms of cost-effectiveness and consumer outcomes.

Key Point: Given the results and conclusions of recent meta-analyses and the need to apply the evidence in favour of CHF-MP's to best serve the health care system and those affected, there is an urgent need to perform a head-to-head comparison of clinic *vs.* home-based CHF management.

RESEARCH OBJECTIVES

The *WHICH? Trial* will play an essential role in *translating research into practice* by determining the actual cost and benefits (both in terms of the health care system and the consumer perspective) of applying both forms of clinic and home-based CHF-MP to the more than 50,000 patients in metropolitan regions throughout Australia discharged from hospital with CHF each year. Furthermore, it will determine which one of these two forms of CHF-MP is most worthy of funding to meet the needs of the health care system and affected individuals. In order to achieve our objectives, we propose to undertake a multi-centre, randomized controlled study of these two forms of CHF-MP to determine which is most cost-effective in applying gold-standard pharmacotherapy and improving unacceptably high morbidity/mortality rates. It will test the following hypothesis:

In typically older patients with CHF exposed to a multidisciplinary, home-based CHF-MP in the 12 months following an acute hospitalisation, there will be no difference in:

1) The combined cost of hospital & community-based health care
2) Patient/consumer quality of life (*co-primary endpoint*)

As compared to a similar multidisciplinary CHF-MP applied via a specialist CHF outpatient clinic.

STUDY DESIGN OF THE WHICH? TRIAL

The schema below [Figure 7.8] shows the key features of the *WHICH? Trial*: a multi-centre, randomised study with independent teams at each site randomised to provide clinic or home-based intervention. Overall, this study is designed to provide appropriate study power, minimise interventional contamination and operator bias in addition to providing blinded assessment of study endpoints.

METHODS

Patient cohort & selection criteria: All patients admitted to the following tertiary-referral hospitals (responsible clinician) in four States will be screened for the presence of CHF:

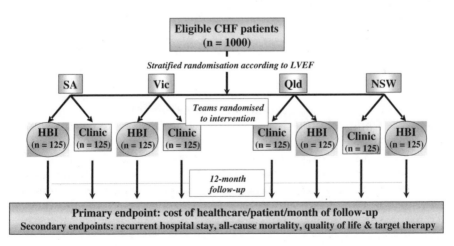

Figure 7.8. Key features of the WHICH? Trial

- The Queen Elizabeth Hospital, Adelaide, South Australia (Prof. John Horowitz)
- The Alfred Hospital, Melbourne, Victorial (Prof. Henry Krum)
- St George Hospital, Sydney, New South Wales (Assoc. Prof. Davidson)
- The Prince Alexandra Hospital, Brisbane, Queensland (Prof. Tom Marwick)

Data from the **BENCH Study** of all CHF-MP's in Australia [9] (see Application no. 1 above) confirm that all of these sites routinely screen patients for CHF to enter pre-existing programs of care and manage 200 – 300 CHF patients per annum. Study targets for patient recruitment are, therefore, entirely feasible. Selection criteria are based on the working definition of CHF proposed by the new NHF Guidelines written by Prof's Krum and Stewart [6] and that applied in many CHF-MP's around the world [10]:

Patients admitted to these four institutions will be invited to participate in the study if they are aged ≥55 years, to be discharged to home, have an underlying diagnosis of CHF with related persistent moderate to severe symptoms and a history of ≥1 admission for acute heart failure.

Patient recruitment and follow-up: 1000 patients (250 from each centre) will be recruited over an 18-month period from these four tertiary centres and subject to 2 months follow-up

Clinic versus home-based CHF-MP's: It is important to note that it would be unethical to randomise patients to *usual care* not involving a CHF-MP [6]. Consistent with literature and established CHF-MP's [8, 10], both intervention groups will incorporate the key components of care outlined below:

Multidisciplinary approach	Close link with primary care
Careful assessment of risk	Early warning systems
Gold-standard pharmacology &	Promotion of self-care strategies
non-pharmacological strategies [6]	Holistic/individualised care

For each CHF patient, a core team comprising a specially trained heart failure nurse, their hospital physician, a pharmacist with specialist advice/support from a dedicated cardiologist at each hospital will guide their management (dedicated team for each form of intervention). Regardless of the form of intervention, the patient's GP will retain a key role in their subsequent management. Additional support/health care will be provided by community-based pharmacists, community nurses, domiciliary care and social workers as determined by the patient's individual needs and using current funding initiatives in primary care.

The two arms of the study will fundamentally differ in terms of the *focus and location* of the specialist CHF management. In the **clinic model**, patients are required to attend the specialist clinic located at the tertiary referral centre which acts as a focal point for specialist care. In the *home-based model*, there is a strong focus on managing the patient in the community.

Key Point: There are potentially important differences between these two approaches relating to: 1) cost of application, 2) impact on morbidity and mortality, 3) attainment of gold-standard management, 4) patient self-care and 5) the patient's (and carer's) quality of life.

STUDY ENDPOINTS

The *WHICH Trial* is appropriately designed to determine clinically significant differences in respect to the above outcomes between these two forms of CHF-MP's. A health economic analysis (to be undertaken by Assoc/Prof. Scuffham) will compare the *cost-benefits* of the clinic and home-based approach on the basis of potential cost-savings in reducing recurrent admissions and validated *quality of life* instruments applied to monitor patient-orientated outcomes. Significantly, the overall results of this study and potentially important disparities between potential cost-savings and quality of life will be carefully analysed by an independent panel of expert clinicians, health care policy makers and administrators and patients (and carers) with CHF.

Key Point: The **WHICH Trial** has the potential to identify a model of care that will derive annual savings of at least $400,000 and 1,800 fewer days of hospital stay per 1000 CHF patients treated.

RESEARCH TEAM

The experienced *WHICH? Trial* research team has a strong collaborative history * that will enable it to not only undertake the research study as proposed, but also ensure that the results of this vitally important study are translated in real-life to not only improve health outcomes in relation to one of Australia's most important public health issues, but achieve these in the most cost-efficient and consumer friendly manner possible.

NB. All of the research team have collaborated on nationally competitive research projects. *

Importantly, as can be appreciated by the list below, the research team represents the interests and expertise of cardiovascular nursing, cardiology, health economics, health policy and consumers. In this respect, Prof. Simon Stewart is an international expert in pioneering and applying CHF-MP's. He also has strong links to the Heart Foundation (policy advice). Prof. Henry Krum is an international expert in CHF and clinical trials. In collaboration with Prof. Stewart, he has written the NHF updated guidelines for its gold-standard management [6]. Assoc/Prof. Paul Scuffham is an internationally renowned health-economist. Prof's Tom Marwick and John Horowitz are internationally renowned academic cardiologists. Assoc/Prof. Trish Davidson is a national expert in CHF nursing and chronic disease management and Prof. Claire Jackson is a national leader in general practice/primary care. All of these investigators have strong track records in undertaking internationally competitive research and translating such research into clinical practice. The team also includes Mr Tony Wade a highly experienced and nationally renowned consumer advocate who will coordinate consumer views and participation and Prof. Andrew Wilson from Queensland Health who will provide expert advice from a health administrative perspective. Ms. Andrea Driscoll is an NHMRC funded PhD candidate who has undertaken the NHF-funded BENCH Study involving 60 CHF-MP's and 1000 Australian CHF patients will provide expert advice to the study.

GOVERNANCE AND RESEARCH CAPACITY

As indicated above, the senior investigators listed above have extensive experience in under-taking large-scale clinical research. Prof. Stewart will coordinate a management team (including a dedicated study coordinator and Prof's Krum and Assoc/Prof Scuffham) to ensure that all management teams (two at each site) are applying the same principles and standards of care and following study protocols in addition to acquiring high quality study data. As indicated in the list of participating sites, a dedicated investigator will be responsible for supervising patient recruitment and follow-up at each site. Data collection and analysis will be centrally coordinated by Prof. Stewart's research team at the University of South Australia with assistance of key personnel from Monash University (Prof. Krum's CCRE in Heart Failure) and University of Queensland (Prof Stewart's Care & Prevention of Heart Disease Research Unit).

BUDGET RELATIVE TO VALUE FOR MONEY

Each of the collaborating centres has the current capacity to provide two parallel forms of CHF-MP (i.e. two independent teams) with funding for key personnel (particularly a dedicated specialist heart failure nurse). The **WHICH? TRIAL** predominantly requires personnel to coordinate and collect data at each centre in addition to an overall coordinator. Considering that CHF contributes to more than **$1 billion in health care** costs per annum with a preventable component of at least **$100 million in hospital care per annum**, the cost of this study (approximately $900,000) represents extremely good value for money. Regardless of the ultimate comparisons between hospital and clinic-based care, this study will provide vital data for the sustainable funding of CHF-MP's throughout Australia's metropolitan regions; the approximately 25% of CHF patients living in rural and remote Australia often require alternative models of care [6]). Importantly it will inform policy decisions on the relative cost of systematically applying CHF-MP's from the Federal and State government funding perspective while ensuring that the needs of consumers/carers are considered.

REFERENCES

1. Stewart S, *et al. Eur J Heart Failure* 2002; 4: 361–71.
2. Stewart S, *et al. Eur J Heart Failure* 2001; 3: 315–322.
3. Krum H & Stewart S. *Med J Aust* 2006; 184: 147–148.
4. Krum H *et al. Med J Aust* 2001; 174: 439–444
5. Abhayaratna WP, *et al. Med J Aust* 2006; 184: 151–154
6. *CSANZ/NHF Guidelines for the Prevention, Detection & Management of People with CHF in Australia.*
7. Murphy N, *et al. Eur Heart J* – Accepted Aug 2005
8. McAllister F, *et al. J Am Coll Cardiol* 2004; 44: 810–19.*
9. Driscoll A, *et al. Eur J Cardiovascular Nursing.* 2006; 5: 75–82.
10. Stewart S & Blue L. *Specialist Nurse Intervention in Chronic Heart Failure.* BMJ Books 2004.

DEVELOPING A COMPELLING CURRICULUM VITAE

Consistent with the importance of developing a compelling research application that will give you the best possible chance of funding success, it is vitally important for you to compose (and then maintain with each 'success') a compelling curriculum vitae. In a busy research environment, this document will be needed in a variety of guises, from the full version required for employment and fellowship applications to abbreviated/'highlight' versions for grant applications, research reports and public forums. It makes sense to put some strategic thoughts and energy into constructing a 'master' document that will grow in size as your career progresses. Even otherwise 'empty' sections can serve as a stimulus for attaining greater things, such as having a section entitled 'Invited Presentations – International Conferences'. This master document can then be modified to suit any purpose, as suggested above, to provide a simple one or two-page résumé that highlights your key attributes.

Naturally, like most human endeavours, there is a plethora of opinion with respect to developing a 'winning' curriculum vitae (a Latin term literally meaning 'the course of one's life'). The text box provides a list of websites that offer advice on this subject.

Useful Internet sites for CV writing*

Winning CVs:
http://www.winning-cvs.co.uk/cvtips.htm
Putting together an effective CV:
http://www.prospects.ac.uk/cms/ShowPage/Home_page/Applications_
    and_interviews/Applications/Compiling_a_CV/p!eXfdpk
Your PhD . . . What next?:
http://www.prospects.ac.uk/cms/ShowPage/Home_page/Your_PhD____
    what_next_/p!edabXF
Writing an Impressive Curriculum Vitae (CV):
http://www.hr.lanl.gov/FindJob/writing-cv.shtml
Writing a Curriculum Vitae for Research Proposals and Grant
    Applications:
http://ccnr.ntu.edu.au/research6.html
Resume Writing Tips for Preparing A Curriculum Vitae:
http://www.free-resume-tips.com/resumetips/curriclm.html
Curriculum Vitae:
http://purdue.placementmanual.com/resume/resume-14.html
Presenting your PhD in CVs and applications:
http://www.grad.ac.uk/cms/ShowPage/Home_page/Online_resources/Just_
    for_Postgrads/Marketing_yourself_to_employers/Presenting_your_
    PhD_in_CVs_and_applications/p!eXecffm

* All accessed September 2006

The following list represents a summary of the key areas of advice provided by these sites:

- A well written curriculum vitae 'paints a picture' of you that will match your skills and achievements as well as your future ambitions.
- The curriculum vitae should be typed and set out in a logical and easy-to-read format, with pages numbered.
- Focus on your positives and if 'compelled' to list areas of weakness (e.g. stating how many times your book has made it to the *New York Times* Bestseller list!), wherever possible, turn that weakness into the strength ('appropriate to the nature of my research, I have focussed on publishing my research in professional journals and producing policy reports that have made a substantive impact on healthcare delivery').

- Always check and double-check your curriculum vitae or application form for spelling errors and punctuation.
- The way you present information on your curriculum vitae is relatively flexible and will depend on what you have to offer. However, it is generally recognised that all curriculum vitae tend to include the following sections:
  - personal details
  - personal profile/career objective
  - education
  - experience
  - positions of responsibility/achievements/interests
  - referees
- At a more specific level, a research-focused curriculum vitae would include a combination of the following:
  - research interests/areas of expertise
  - PhD thesis
  - publications
  - scientific presentations or conferences attended
  - competitive and non-competitive funding
  - professional memberships
  - fellowships and awards
  - teaching/mentoring and administrative experiences
- Prioritizing your top skills and experience to be presented in the first or uppermost section of your curriculum vitae makes sense. Then provide additional details relating to educational, employment or academic experience.

In the spirit of a 'warts and all' examination of my own philosophy and approach to presenting a curriculum vitae (it is worth noting that I change the format annually in line with a new background for my Powerpoint presentations!), the following is a mini-version of my curriculum vitae. Once again, it is up to the reader to judge whether this represents a good, bad or indifferent one!

CURRICULUM VITAE

Name:	**PROFESSOR SIMON STEWART**
Position:	**Head of the Preventative Cardiology Unit** **Baker Heart Research Institute**
Contact Address:	PO Box 6492, St Kilda Road Central, Melbourne, Victoria, Australia, 3008
Phone/Fax:	+61 (0)43 8302 111 / +618 3 8532 1100
E-mail:	simon.stewart@baker.edu.au

Honorary Titles: Fellow of the American Heart Association (FAHA)

Nurse Fellow of the European Society of Cardiology (NFESC)

Fellow of the Cardiac Society of Australia & New Zealand (FCANZ)

Adjunct Appointments: Professor, School of Medicine
University of Adelaide, South Australia

Professor, School of Nursing
Deakin University, Melbourne, Victoria

Professor, Nethersole School of Nursing
Chinese University Hong Kong, Hong Kong

Professor, Department of Medicine
University of the Witwatersrand, South Africa

Professor, Preventative Medicine & Epidemiology
Monash University, Melbourne, Victoria

Qualifications

1996–1999 **Doctor of Philosophy**, '*Optimising therapeutic efficacy in acute and chronic cardiac disease states*', Department of Medicine, Adelaide University, South Australia

1992–1993 **Graduate Diploma of Adult Education**, University of South Australia, South Australia

1991–1992 **Bachelor of Nursing**, Flinders University, South Australia

1990–1991 **Intensive Therapy Unit Certificate**, The Queen Elizabeth Hospital, South Australia

1985–1988 **Registered Nurse**, The Queen Elizabeth Hospital, South Australia

1981–1984 **Bachelor of Arts**, University of Adelaide, South Australia

Employment

2006–Present **Head of the Preventative Cardiology Unit:** Baker Heart Research Unit, Melbourne, Victoria, Australia

2004–2006 **Professor of Health Research:** Faculty of Health Sciences (School of Medicine), University of Queensland, Brisbane, Australia

2002–2006	**National Heart Foundation of Australia/Roche Chair of Cardiovascular Nursing:** The School of Nursing and Midwifery, Division of Health Sciences, University of South Australia, Adelaide, Australia
2001–2002	**NHMRC Career Development Award: Associate Research Professor of Cardiovascular Nursing:** The School of Nursing and Midwifery, Division of Health Sciences, University of South Australia, Adelaide, Australia
1996–1999	**National Heart Foundation of Australia Post-graduate Research Scholar:** Department of Medicine, University of Adelaide, Adelaide, South Australia
1999–2001	**National Heart Foundation of Australia Ralph Reader Fellow:** British Heart Foundation CRI in Heart Failure, University of Glasgow, Scotland
1993–1996	**Senior Cardiac Research Nurse:** Department of Cardiology, The Queen Elizabeth Hospital/University of Adelaide, South Australia
1991–1992	**Nurse Educator:** School of Nursing, The Queen Elizabeth Hospital, South Australia
1988–1991	**Registered Nurse:** The Queen Elizabeth Hospital, Woodville, South Australia
1985–1988	**Student Registered Nurse:** The Queen Elizabeth Hospital, South Australia

Publications

Published Articles in Peer-Reviewed Journals

- **Refereed Research Publications: <u>Highly cited</u>**
  1. **Stewart S**, Horowitz JD. Home-based intervention in congestive heart failure: long-term implications on readmission and survival. *Circulation* 2002; 105: 2861–2866 [**IF = 11.6**] + [**65**]

- **Refereed Research Publications: <u>Top Clinical Journals</u>**
  2. Pearson S, Inglis S, McLennan S, Brennan L, Russell M, Wilkinson M, Thompson DR, **Stewart S**. Prolonged effects of a home-based intervention in patients with chronically illness. *Archives of Internal Medicine* 2006; 166: 645–650 [**IF = 8.0**] + [**1**]

- **Refereed Research Publications: <u>Specialist Journals</u>**
  3. Clark RA, Yallop J, Wickett D, Krum H, Tonkin A, **Stewart S**. Nursing sans frontières: a three year case study of multistate registration to support nursing practice using information technology. *Australian Journal of Advanced Nursing* Sep–Nov 2006; 24(1): 39–45.

- **Reviews and Editorials: <u>Top Clinical Journals</u>**
  4. McMurray JJV, **Stewart S**. Chilling findings: The need for winter vigilance in heart failure (Editorial). *Journal Cardiac Failure* 2006; 12: 120–121 [**IF = 2.9**]

- **Reviews and Editorials: <u>Specialist Journals</u>**
  5. Davidson PM, Worrall-Carter L, Finn JC, **Stewart S** on behalf of the Australian Network for Cardiovascular Nursing Research. Beyond competition: a new paradigm for collaborative cardiovascular research in Australia (Editorial). *European Journal of Cardiovascular Nursing* 2006; 4: 181–182

- **Books**
  1. **Stewart S**, Inglis S, Hawkes. *Chronic Cardiac Care: A Practical Guide to Specialist Nurse Management*, 2006, BMJ Books (Blackwell Publishing Group), London

- **Book Chapters (other than those published in self-edited books)**
  1. *Heart failure handbook*. McMurray JJV, Berry C and O'Meara E (editors). Science Press Ltd, London (in press): **Stewart** S, Non-pharmacological therapy & multidisciplinary management

- **Major Reports**
  1. Krum H, Jelinek M, **Stewart S**, Sindone A, Atherton J, Hawkes A on behalf of the National Heart Foundation of Australia and Cardiac Society of Australia and New Zealand Chronic Heart Failure Clinical Practice Guidelines Expert Writing Panel. *Guidelines for the Prevention, Detection and Management of People with Chronic Heart Failure in Australia* (2006)

Peer-Reviewed Abstract Presentations at International Meetings

XXVI Congress of the European Society of Cardiology & World Congress of Cardiology, Barcelona, Spain (September 2006)
1. Ultimate cost–benefits of altering the natural history of chronic heart failure via multidisciplinary, home-based intervention: Ten-year follow-up of typically old and fragile patients. Inglis S, Horowitz JD, **Stewart S**

Invited Presentations at International Meetings

55th Annual Scientific Meeting of the Cardiac Society of Australia and New Zealand. Canberra, Australia (August 2006)
1. *KEY NOTE ADDRESS*: Talking to our patients again: Back to the future for cardiovascular nurses? (*Inaugural Cardiovascular Nursing Lecture – Annual Address at the CSANZ meeting*)

Summary of Current National/International Competitive Funding

INVESTIGATORS	TITLE	DATES	FUNDS	SOURCE
Askew, Wilkinson, **Stewart,** Dick, Schrader, Wade, Marwick, Scuffham, Jackson, McFarlane	Detection and management of depression in general practice patients with chronic manifestations of ischaemic heart disease	2006–2008	2006 $A202,185, 2007 $A188,450, 2008 $A109,163	NH&MRC General Practice Clinical Research Grants

Competitive Scholarships/Fellowships

National Health and Medical Research Council of Australia, Public Health Postgraduate Medical Research Scholarship for Ms Sally Inglis (**$78,000**) *Principal Supervisor*

Previous Competitive Research Grants

Principal Applicant/Investigator
Diabetes Australia Research Grant (2004), 12-month grant for the DATA Study (**$40,000**)

Non-Competitive Research Grants/Support

Principal or Co-applicant
Adcock Ingram, Republic of South Africa (2006), three-year sponsorship of the 'Heart of Soweto' Study
(**R 2 million–$460,000**)

Professional Activities: International Societies

Cardiac Society of Australia and New Zealand

- Named Annual Lecture to commence in at 2006 Scientific Meeting
- Inaugural Secretary of the Heart Failure Working Group (2003–to date)
- Member of the Organising Committee of the Annual Scientific Meeting (Adelaide – 1997 & 2003)
- Fellow (2005–to date)
- Member (2000–2004)
- Affiliate Member (1993–1999)

Professional Activities: Significant Achievements

The American Heart Association

- Awarded Best Poster Presentation in the 'popular science' section at the 2000 Scientific Meeting in New Orleans
- Selected as the *first ever* non-US-based nurse to be awarded the Council on Cardiovascular Nursing's Best Research Article of the Year Award (2000)
- Selected as the *first ever* non-US-based nurse to be awarded an International Fellowship of the Council on Cardiovascular Nursing (2000)
- Selected as the *first ever* non-US-based nurse to be awarded the Cardiovascular Nursing Council's Martha Hill New Investigator Award (1999)

Professional Activities: International Peer-Review Journals

- **Editor**

European Journal of Cardiovascular Nursing (2002–2006): An official journal of the European Society of Cardiology

- **Associate Editor**

International Journal of Cardiology (2006–to date)

- **Issue Editor**

October 2001 issue of the *Journal of Cardiovascular Nursing – International perspectives*

- **Editorial Board Member**

Journal of Cardiovascular Nursing (2000–to date)

- **Peer Reviewer**

European Heart Journal (1998–to date)

Professional Activities: Expert Consultancy

National Institute of Clinical Studies (Commonwealth Government of Australia)

- Member of the Organising Committee for Heart Failure 2004 Meeting
- Invited member of an Expert Panel on measuring the burden of heart failure in Australia (Sydney, August 2002)
- Member of the Expert Panel on heart failure targets in Australia
- Expert consultant – key targets in the treatment and management of heart failure (2001)

International Research Links

The University of the Witwatersrand, South Africa

Professor Karen Sliwa-Hahnle: the *Heart of Soweto Study* a large epidemiologic research programme involving more than 15,000 men and women from Soweto in South Africa that will address the following hypotheses:

1. The profound political and socio-economic changes in South Africa have negatively impacted on the cardiovascular risk behaviour profile and subsequent incidence of heart disease.
2. An increasing incidence of HIV, compounded by the recent introduction of anti-retroviral therapy, is associated with a parallel increase in acute myocardial infarction due to thromboembolic events.
3. Culturally specific programmes focussed on primary/secondary prevention and chronic disease management initially based at Baragwaneth Hospital and extending to nurse-led community centres throughout Soweto will improve the risk factor profile and cardiac-related outcomes in that community.*

Summary of Career Highlights

- *World First Appointment*

World first appointment as National Heart Foundation Chair of Cardiovascular Nursing (University of South Australia) in 2002–2006.

- *Honorary Appointments*

Professorial appointments at prestigious international universities in Asia and Africa in addition to similar appointments at prestigious Australian institutions. Fellow of the American Heart Association, Inaugural Nurse Fellow of the European Society of Cardiology and the only nurse to be awarded Fellowship of the Cardiac Society of Australia & New Zealand.

- *Publications*

Published eight books via international publishers, with more than 20,000 copies sold. In the past five years, published more than 60 research reports in high-ranking medical journals – including 30 epidemiologic reports (average impact factor of journal >5.0 in both cases).

- *Invited Presentations*

Presented more than 50 invited lectures at prestigious international conferences on the role of chronic cardiac disease management, cost implications of cardiovascular disease and its management and epidemiology of chronic cardiac disease states.

- *Research Funding*

Current research funding worth more than $AU 6 million. Continuously funded by the National Heart Foundation and National Health & Medical Research Council of Australia for the past 10 years.

- *Research Supervision*

Currently supervising 5 PhD candidates with nationally competitive research scholarships: remainder funded by locally competitive research scholarships.

- *Expert Roles*

Past Chair of the Heart Foundation's Research Grant in Aid Committee (2003–2005), member of a number of prestigious national committees, peer reviewer for high-impact medical journals (e.g. *Lancet* and *Circulation*), editor *European Journal of Cardiovascular Nursing*, editorial board member of the *European Journal of Heart Failure* and member of the inaugural board of the newly formed World Society of Heart Failure (Chair of Nursing Panel).

- *Career Highlights*

First nurse to be awarded an NHF Postgraduate Research Scholarship, winner of the prestigious NHF Ralph Reader Overseas Scholarship, winner of the AHA's Martha Hill New Investigator Award, Young Tall Poppy Award and Inaugural winner of an NH&MRC Career Development Award with supplementary support.

COMPLETING A SUCCESSFUL INTERVIEW

Whilst it is possible to fully control a written application and therefore present to peer reviews the exact information you want to them, undertaking a competitive interview for either direct research funding or personal support (e.g. a Post-Doctoral Fellowship) is fraught with danger. In this circumstance, it is not the research team or individual that 'controls' the flow of information but the members of the interview panel who will ask probing questions. However, there are a number of highly effective strategies that you can employ to improve your competitiveness relative to those also being interviewed:

- Talk to past members of the same interview panel to determine the usual format and flow of the interview in addition to their impressions of what did and didn't work for those being interviewed.
- Wherever possible, include a senior researcher who has been through a rigorous, competitive research interview (preferably including the same interview process with a positive result).
- Prepare your interview strategy according to your research on what it takes to be successful.
- Practise your interview strategy prior to the actual event.
- If there is a team of researchers being interviewed, carefully manage who will be responsible for what portion of the interview: there is nothing worse than antagonism or confusion between team members.
- If given the opportunity to present your case, prepare it in the same way and as comprehensively as you would a written application, focussing on

being clear and precise and including graphics or handouts to support the message that you are trying to present.

- Be consistent with your original application: do not substantially change your plans without a very good reason.
- Always respond to issues raised by any peer-reviewer comments received prior to the interview.
- Throughout the interview, remain calm and consider your answers carefully and with critical honesty with respect to potential limitations: denial of obvious limitations or critical research issues will undoubtedly antagonise the interview panel.
- Listen when required (avoid the impulse to interrupt panel members) and use positive body language.

It is important to note that with any public presentation, it is not only the quality of the research that counts but the manner in which it is presented. If you are able to convey your passion and excitement about the proposed research or your research career to the interview panel, you are likely to leave them with an indelible and favourable impression that will overcome the usual 'interviewer' fatigue that comes with interviewing so many people. If you are ranked equally with another research team or individual for the quality of research or curriculum vitae, it is quite probable that your ability to remain composed and organised and still convey a passion for your research during the interview process will give you the competitive edge for successful funding. Excellent interviewing skills should, therefore, be added to your list of essential skills that form part of the extensive armoury of attributes of a successful researcher.

SUMMARY

Unless you are able to sell the quality and potential value of your research through the written word and face-to-face communication (this involves more than just your verbal presentation) in an effective manner, you are unlikely to receive competitive funding. As with most activities, it requires practice and experience. In the early phases of your research career, you will benefit from the support and presence of more experienced peers.

Key Points: There are an art and science to completing effective research grant applications and successfully navigating a competitive research interview. Both forms of assessment require extensive preparation, strategic thought, clear and precise presentation and, overall, a sense of passion and excitement to compel the assessment panel to provide you with funding.

---

8 Putting It All Together: A Self-Fulfilling Prophecy of Career Success in Health Research

INTRODUCTION

The basic premise of this book is that it is eminently possible to create a self-fulfilling prophecy of career success in health research through strategic intent, hard work and the support of more experienced researchers with your best interests at heart. Fortunately, not everyone's career goals are the same and the options and pathways to achieve your ultimate goals (that may well evolve over time) are many and varied. It would strike me as futile, however, if someone committed to a career in health research in order to make a tangible 'difference' in an area close to their heart and spent only a few moments thinking about how they are going to get into a position to make that difference – assuming that they have enough vision and self-belief to become an important contributor to human health if they attain a position of seniority and/or influence. Certainly, the personal reflections (later in this chapter) provide a uniform sense of wanting to achieve something beyond fame and money (although this is always nice!!). Hopefully, this book has stimulated you to think more critically about why and how you should pursue a successful career in health research. Throughout, there are a number of key messages that are briefly revisited in this concluding chapter.

PUTTING IT ALL TOGETHER

Rather than repeat in detail the strategies outlined in the previous chapters, this chapter is designed to provide a final checklist of eight critical questions (and related ancillary questions) for the emerging health researcher to consider with respect to contemplating how to build a successful career:

1. **How can I plan strategically for a successful career in health research?**
   a. Do I have vision for the future of a successful career in health research?

   b. Am I aware of the strategic milestones typically attained by successful researchers during their career?

   c. What can I do to make myself competitive even prior to formally commencing my career in health research?

   d. Who are the senior researchers most likely to offer me the opportunity to develop a research career and provide quality and supportive mentorship/supervision?

   e. Who are my immediate peers, what are their initial experiences in attempting to similarly develop a research career and how can we support each other in our mutual goals?

   f. Am I still professionally active and committed to assisting the overall goals of my health discipline through my combined expertise in clinical practice, research and education?

2. Do I currently have the skills and knowledge to become an expert health researcher?

   a. What are my strengths?

   b. What are my weaknesses?

   c. What miscellaneous/ancillary skills do I need to develop?

   d. What strategies do I need to apply to give myself a career-long advantage?

3. Who are my competitors and how have they achieved success?

   a. What is the benchmark for research success in my health discipline?

   b. What is my threshold for personal success and how much higher is it relative to current benchmarks?

   c. What strategies do my competitors and peers use to achieve success?

4. What research topic will sustain a research career?

   a. What is the likely impact of my research in terms of better health outcomes, publications and my personal career goals?

   b. Who else is active in this research?

   c. Which research team would best suit my research interests and career goals?

   d. What is the natural evolution of my current research interests?

   e. What skills and knowledge domains do I need to become an expert in this field?

5. What are the essential building blocks of a successful research career?

   a. Am I prepared to undertake a full-time PhD?

   b. Do I have a strategic plan for my PhD to ensure it is completed in a productive and timely manner?

   c. Do my PhD supervisors have my best interests at heart and have a strategic plan for my future career?

   d. Am I planning early for a post-doctoral research fellowship?

   e. Which post-doctoral institution and research team will best suit my future research plans?

6. What strategies will enable me to become a prolific publisher?
a. How can I improve my writing skills?
b. What strategies will improve my publication output?
c. What are the most prestigious journals relevant to my area of research and what type of studies/reviews are accepted for publication?
d. Are there any opportunities to contribute to book chapters and/or publish my own book (e.g. based on my PhD thesis)?

7. How can I successfully apply for competitive research funds?
a. How can I improve the quality of my research applications and my interview skills?
b. How do successful researchers apply for competitive research funds?
c. Do I have the support of experienced researchers to assist me in the process?
d. Have I created a 'winning' record to assist me in applying for funding to support the next phase of my research career?
e. Have I consistently outperformed my peers in terms of quality and quantity?

8. Am I presenting myself in the best possible light?
a. How can I improve my curriculum vitae to best highlight my strengths?
b. Am I fully prepared for a searching interview with answers to the most likely questions? (e.g. what are your strengths and weaknesses?)
c. Do I have a positive and negative attitude?
d. Am I demonstrating my passion and commitment for my area of research in every aspect of my activities?

PERSONAL REFLECTIONS ON AN EMERGING RESEARCH CAREER

Given that this book has been largely focussed on a 'Simon Stewart-centric' approach to career enhancement and development in the field of health research, it makes sense to provide some external influence and perspective to balance the ledger. This section of the book, therefore, comprises some personal reflections from a diverse group of researchers from a range of health disciplines who are either enrolled for a PhD or have made the transition to an early post-doctoral position. It is worth noting, of course, that each of these researchers has a close connection to my research programme. These reflections have only been subject to minor editing and all individuals are strong-willed individuals who are unafraid to voice their opinions.

As part of this exercise, a total of 14 early career researchers (with a 93 per cent response rate) were asked to respond to the following topics in whatever way they wished:

1. a brief personal/background biography;
2. a snap-shot of where you are at in your research careers;
3. the major factors that you see underpin success;
4. the major hurdles;
5. what you hope to achieve.

As the majority of these successful researchers are female (there is only one male to add to my male perspective!), it is worth (briefly) considering the particular issues faced by 'women in research'. Some key quotes from a recent report from Monash University in Australia, entitled 'When Research Works for Women' (Dever M, Morrison Z, Dalton B and Tayton S (2006) Monash University, Melbourne, ISBN 0-9756822-1-0, p ii), resonate with many of the issues touched upon in the following reflections from a broad range of female academics:

'There are other measures of success in that I also feel successful in the sense of having been able to launch other people's careers or have a role to play in nurturing the next generation of researchers.'

'I had a very productive postdoc where I got some big papers out and the whole advantage of that is that it sets you up for getting a position back here.'

'I took full advantage of what was available, I made sure that I got papers prepared for conferences, I went to overseas conferences every year, the local conference whenever there was one and they supported me in that respect.'

'I think we sometime make too much of the interruption of children and sure, they interrupt you, but they also provide you with an incredible balance and perspective on life.'

PERSONAL REFLECTION 1: JAN CAMERON, PhD STUDENT, SCHOOL OF NURSING, DEAKIN UNIVERSITY, BURWOOD, VICTORIA, AUSTRALIA

PERSONAL BACKGROUND

I am an experienced nurse clinician with post-graduate qualifications in cardiovascular nursing and health education and promotion. My expert skills are in the management of patients with heart failure and in 2001 I helped to establish a heart failure management programme. During this time, I have become acutely aware of the barriers that patients encounter in undertaking self-care behaviours. With this in mind, I began PhD research in 2004 to further investigate barriers to self-care, in particular the impact of cognitive impairment. I was awarded a prestigious scholarship from NHMRC/NHF in 2005 that has enabled me to undertake the research full time.

RESEARCH

A pilot study was undertaken to examine the relationship between heart failure self-care and mild cognitive impairment. This has been the first study that attempted to correlate CHF self-care using a tool that measures the decision-making process to manage the symptoms of ankle swelling and difficulty breathing that are common to this syndrome (Riegel *et al.*, 2004) whilst at the same time measuring the cognitive domains of memory recall, orientation, attention, calculation, language and visual construction from the Mini Mental State Examination (Tombaugh and McIntyre, 1992). Although the study did not find the anticipated correlation between lower levels of self-care and lower levels of cognitive function, it has taken me on quite a different research path than originally planned. Future research is to be conducted to validate the use of both the clinical instruments to screen patients in order to determine those who may be competent self-managers and those who may not be. Ultimately, it is anticipated that this knowledge may help formulate a screening tool that can help nurses predict the intensity of support and follow-up required in order for poor self-managers to remain out of hospital.

SUCCESS

There are three major factors that I perceive to underpin success in conducting the research programme:

1. Supervisors
   These need to be carefully chosen. They need to have an excellent grounding in the particular research field, be able to provide constructive and timely feedback, be able to support your development as a researcher and be politically astute in furthering your career progression.
2. Support from elsewhere
   A collaborative group of research colleagues that are mentors, friends and confidants can help pull you through the dire times and help develop your writing and publishing skills. Moral support from family and friends help to keep you sane.
3. The research environment
   A partnership between the university and hospital where the research is being conducted makes life easier. Research schools which are conducted regularly by both the university and supervisors help in your research development.

MAJOR HURDLES

- Time management – it can be very frustrating when your supervisors cannot meet agreed time plans and this requires the student to be flexible and re-set their own time frames.

- Getting published – having manuscripts rejected by peer-reviewed journals can be soul-destroying. Getting that first published article with your name as the first author is something to celebrate.
- Coping with the unexpected – this can come in two forms. Supervisors may give only short notice to complete a written submission that can help further your career. Additionally, there are things beyond our control and life can place many unexpected burdens which can include overcoming a major health illness at the most inopportune time.

WHAT I HOPE TO ACHIEVE

- To complete a major piece of research that has relevance to CHF clinical nursing practice
- To have professional recognition as an expert in understanding barriers to CHF self-care

REFERENCES

Riegel B, Carlson B, Moser D, Seburn M, Hicks F and Roland V (2004) Psychometric testing of The Self-Care of Heart Failure Index. *Journal of Cardiac Failure* 10(4): 350–360.
Tombaugh T and McIntyre N (1992) The Mini-Mental State Examination: A comprehensive review. *Journal of American Geriatric Society* 40: 922–935.

PERSONAL REFLECTION 2: SKYE MCLENNAN, PhD STUDENT, SCHOOL OF PSYCHOLOGY, UNIVERSITY OF ADELAIDE, SOUTH AUSTRALIA, AUSTRALIA

A SLOW START

I am a 30-year-old female who is in the very early stages of her research career. I completed a degree in an allied health discipline around two years ago, with the intention of establishing myself as a clinician. Although I had always wanted to do university-level teaching, I did not have a clear idea of how to break into this area, and had not even considered a career in research. This lack of knowledge was my main barrier to forging a career in research. I did not have direct contact with anyone who had created a research career. If any of my lecturers was significantly involved in research, this was not obvious to me. Without any background understanding, I did not know the right questions to ask to determine what I should do. The general advice I was given was that a PhD and some work experience would help in my pursuit.

When a vacancy came up for a part-time research assistant, I grabbed the opportunity. It happened to be in the school of nursing – a discipline not closely related to my own. I worked in the position for around a year, doing low-level tasks under close supervision. Eventually, another opportunity arose for a research position elsewhere in the same school, with the potential for increased responsibility. In this new position, my supervisor could see the benefit, to us both, of my pursuing a research career. He shared some of his insights into the criteria by which researchers are judged, and highlighted the importance of building up a publication portfolio, attending national and international conferences to develop professional contacts, and volunteering on a committee (at a junior level). I was also exposed to the processes of applying for grants and funding, and could finally see how a career in research might develop, and I now understood how I could start this process. Around 12 months ago, I eventually enrolled in a PhD. I enrolled in a university with a strong research focus, and through formal workshops within the division, the university disseminated much of the same advice as my previous employer had.

SOURCES OF SUPPORT

A PhD has the potential to be a long and lonely slog; it can also be disempowering because it is often hard to judge the quality and progress of your work. The topic I chose to study was a relatively new area of research, and spanned two disciplines, so it was difficult to find a supervisor (or preferably two or three supervisors) with: adequate content knowledge, adequate commitment and time for supervision, and a personal approach and communication style that meshed well enough with my own to allow us to work closely for at least three years. It took me quite a few months to get a team together that I was happy with, but, in retrospect, I am glad I persisted because I have seen that the quality of supervision makes a huge difference to the ultimate success of the PhD.

In addition to my supervisors, my peers have been invaluable in my success thus far. I was fortunate in my previous research job to have had the opportunity to work within a multidisciplinary team of researchers at different points in their careers. I was able to collaborate on different projects, which provided the opportunity for co-authorship, and exposure to a range of different methodologies. I was able to observe other members of the team go through the various processes of formatting manuscripts for publication, putting together posters for conferences, and compiling applications for scholarships, post docs and study grants, etc. This gave me insight into how to go about these tasks at the ground level, and gave me access to a wider base of mentoring, critique, encouragement and support. Although the formal research group has now broken up, I remain in close contact, and continue to collaborate on research and exchange advice across institutions.

IMPORTANCE OF PROFESSIONAL ACTIVITIES

Based on the experience of my peers and the advice of my mentors, I view the three or four years of PhD candidature as a time to build up a repertoire of skills and experience that will put me in a competitive position by the time I graduate – the actual PhD manuscript is only half the job. To this end, I have participated in a number of different activities on a part-time basis, including:

- working part time as a clinician;
- contributing to research in addition to my PhD project (sometimes paid, and sometimes on a voluntarily or reciprocal basis for my peers);
- co-authoring papers (with my peers, my supervisors, and previous employer);
- presenting work at conferences;
- attending professional interest group meetings;
- volunteering as a student member on professional committees;
- reviewing manuscripts for a journal;
- teaching undergraduate subjects;
- enrolling in university-funded workshops.

These activities are time-consuming, so it has been important to continuously check that the PhD timeline is still on track. However, they are also rewarding, have helped to build my confidence, and have broken the monotony of the PhD. I have consciously looked for these opportunities. I have applied for or enquired about everything that looks interesting or useful, with the anticipation that I will be knocked back on many occasions. I have come to realise that success breeds success. Even a small achievement can open the door for something else. These activities have contributed to my success in winning a nationally competitive scholarship, and a couple of student prizes.

BARRIERS AND FACILITATORS OF SUCCESS SO FAR

So, on reflection, the major hurdles to my success so far have been:

- a lack of knowledge about working in research, and the necessary steps to set up a research career;
- an initial lack of confidence;
- difficulty putting together a supervision team.

The major factors underpinning my success to date have been:

- access to mentoring, advice and support;
- opportunities to participate in research and contribute to publications;
- a willingness to participate in a variety of research-related activities;
- a willingness to take risks and challenge myself (this is much easier with a network of supportive peers and mentors to call on when necessary).

FUTURE AMBITIONS

In the future, I would like to gain an academic post incorporating research as well as some teaching. I definitely want to continue working on multidisciplinary research, as it has been such a rewarding experience so far. I hope to establish myself as an expert in my particular topic area. Beyond this, I do not yet have clear plans. I will continue to use my current approach of looking out for interesting opportunities and see where this leads me.

PERSONAL REFLECTION 3: MARY RUSSELL, PhD CANDIDATE AND LECTURER, SCHOOL OF HEALTH SCIENCES, UNIVERSITY OF SOUTH AUSTRALIA, AUSTRALIA

My research career really began as a newly graduated clinician. Before the days of evidence-based practice, I found myself constantly looking for answers about clinical practice. I wanted to know whether individual cardiac rehabilitation programmes would yield better results than group programmes, and whether the pre-admission clinics led to reduced length of stay and improved outcomes. If not, then I should be spending my time working on other things.

This intellectual curiosity led me to a job as a research therapist in a rehabilitation research unit. The opportunity to work with an experienced research team was a great way to begin developing my experience in a range of research tasks, from recruitment, data gathering and analysis, to writing. During this time, I realised I needed to systematically develop my research knowledge. I enrolled in a Graduate Diploma which included some research courses and a minor research project. The project proved so big that I completed it as a Masters Degree by research. It was a long and challenging experience and a lesson in planning research within the time and resources available. My developing research experience proved to be both valuable and unique in my profession, helping me to secure some great jobs as a senior clinician, manager and academic. Research has been part of my work and professional life for more than a decade since that first research job. Along the way, I was able to build up my curriculum vitae, which included some small research grants, contract research and evaluation, conference presentations, publications and associate supervision of research students.

I am currently working full time in research again, having taken leave from my full-time lecturing job to complete a PhD. Although I had developed considerable experience as a researcher, it became clear to me that if I wanted to develop as an independent and competitive researcher, a doctorate is essential in the contemporary research world. Although I was not an Honours graduate, my research experience, publications and Masters Degree enabled me to secure a PhD place and a highly competitive scholarship. This is one illustration of how gradually developing evidence of research capacity and performance can convince a panel of assessors that you have the potential to move forward as a researcher.

Many people argue that a successful research career, or even a successful doctorate, depends on having a passion for your topic area. While genuine interest and commitment to your research area are important, I believe there are also other keys to success. Intellectual curiosity and the drive to ask and answer questions have enabled me to work on diverse research topics and have sustained me through the ups and downs which are part of research. I have observed that genuine enjoyment of the research process and the desire to keep learning and mastering new aspects of research also set successful researchers apart from the others. Working with mentors can be invaluable in building a research career. In the early days of my research career, a mentor modelled how I could approach difficult tasks like research writing and provided feedback which helped to bring my drafts of grant applications and publications up to an acceptable standard. Since then, mentors have provided valuable encouragement and advice about building my research curriculum vitae by publishing, presenting papers at conferences, undertaking strategic committee work, linking in with successful research teams and undertaking advanced training in research design and data analysis. Most importantly, mentors have encouraged me to take a risk and apply for grants and scholarships in which I did not think I could succeed, been honest about my weaknesses and helped me to see how I could strengthen my applications and research performance. I have also been fortunate to be part of several multidisciplinary research teams and have found the diverse experience and perspectives of my colleagues a great source of critique, expertise and encouragement.

I have also encountered hurdles in developing my research career. The research environment is highly competitive and it is important to develop an attitude of realistically appraising the inevitable knock-backs, while remaining resilient and determined to succeed. It can be hard to break into research. Gaining experience as a research assistant or junior researcher, as I did, was valuable, but it can be difficult to get included in grants, publications and opportunities which are essential to take the next step in building research performance. Lack of formal research training can also be a barrier, but can be overcome by completing relevant coursework and undertaking research training through Honours or a doctoral programme. Research training relies heavily on the role of the supervisor as a teacher, model and mentor, so it is really important to find someone who is willing and available to provide these things throughout your training. I have learnt over many years that there can be a huge difference between having supervisors and having active supervision. Timing can also prove to be an obstacle. There are real advantages to completing a doctorate early in your research and personal life. I have found it challenging to take on one later in my career, when it can be hard to balance a full or part-time commitment to research training against financial, parenting, family and work obligations.

Approaching the end of my doctoral candidacy, I am now thinking about what I hope to achieve in my research career. My mentors have taught me that developing a research track record in the post-doctoral period is essential to developing a research career. My aim is to develop an academic career which involves a minimum of half-time research activity, but also involves research application through teaching, consulting and representation on relevant committees and organisations. Being part of an active and successful research group has shown me that I will need to demonstrate my capacity as a productive researcher, with a track record in a recognised area of relevance to the health of the community. Building a list of quality publications will be essential. Success in obtaining grant funding with other researchers, and in my own right, will be critical to develop from a research trainee to an independent researcher. I envisage that participation as a journal reviewer and committee member, research teaching and developing supervision experience will also be important activities to achieve my goals. I hope that these activities will provide many opportunities to challenge my intellectual curiosity, meet and work with successful researchers and continue to learn and develop as a researcher.

PERSONAL REFLECTION 4: EMILY YORKSTON, FACULTY OF HEALTH SCIENCES, UNIVERSITY OF QUEENSLAND, QUEENSLAND

I had intended to use my undergraduate anatomy and physiology degree as preparation for the graduate medical course. My decision not to follow this career path was based on a number of lifestyle factors. However, I could not see myself fitting the profile of 'researcher' because I was only aware of (and disinterested in) laboratory-based science. A chance offer to undertake a project in injury epidemiology allowed me to discover a scientific research discipline that was not centred on laboratory science and which suited my background and interests in sports and exercise. As I progressed through Honours and then through my PhD, I began to realise that the profile of a scientist can take many forms! As a researcher by chance, I still find it difficult to believe that we are allowed the indulgence of being paid to think!

My research career is in the nubile stage. I have recently submitted my PhD thesis. I was recently awarded a Post-Doctoral Fellowship, which I will use to support my research on a large epidemiological cohort study of nurses and midwives in Australia, New Zealand and the United Kingdom. In this project, I will further develop the analytical and research skills I have learned during my research training. I am now bridging the gap between student and researcher and am building my publications profile, as well as becoming a research higher-degree supervisor.

I believe that success is in equal parts determined by hard work and also by good fortune. I have been privileged to work with a number of talented and driven researchers throughout my career. These mentors have been responsible for helping me to develop core research skills, such as critically appraising my own work and that of others, and have instilled in me the confidence to present and defend the products of my research. I believe that presentation of your work, in scientific journals and in other public forums, is also an essential component of success. Learning and gaining strength from those around you are critical to a successful research career.

Unfortunately, health research is a highly competitive field. To continuously compete against candidates of excellent quality for personal and project funding can be a tiring and demoralising experience. This can be countered by surrounding yourself with colleagues who are encouraging, informed and strategic, and is a valuable way to face the competition head on. Publishing prolifically is also a way to overcome this hurdle.

I have a number of personal and professional goals that I wish to achieve. Maintaining a healthy lifestyle through competitive sport and exercise is exceptionally important to me, and I recognise that the flexibility of an academic research career will allow me to meet this goal.

I am excited to be making the transition from student to fully fledged researcher and to be involved as a colleague with those who have guided me to this point of my career. I would like to make a significant contribution to the discipline of public health and to provide for other researchers the support that my mentors have shown me.

PERSONAL REFLECTION 5: SALLY INGLIS, PhD STUDENT, DIVISION OF HEALTH SCIENCES, UNIVERSITY OF QUEENSLAND, AUSTRALIA

BIOGRAPHY

I really had no idea that I was going to, or that I wanted to, pursue a career in research. Not wanting to make a too specific career choice at an early age or commit myself to spending too long at university, I began my studying with a three-year non-professional, general degree. At the end of my first year at university, I decided that I was unfulfilled by this study and enrolled in second degree at a neighbouring university, which would lead to registration as a health professional. However, I also continued to complete my original degree.

It was at this stage that an early-career researcher, returning from a post-doc overseas, was assigned to mark an assignment I had completed as part of a second-year subject (for my second degree). This chance encounter led to a position as a research assistant (to this early-career researcher) over the coming years as I completed my undergraduate study.

During this time, I developed some preliminary skills in health research. This experience in itself was quite a challenge, it was a whole new world to me and it seemed that everyone else was 10 steps ahead of where I was. There were so many questions I wanted to ask – but I just got on with the job. I think it was this rather unpleasant experience at times (I spent months on end in a windowless room, extracting data from hundreds of dusty files!) which gave me an honest insight into health research and I am glad to say that most projects I have worked on since have been a little more pleasant! Needless to say, I had the opportunity to work with some wonderful mentors and co-researchers, all of whom I am working with currently.

Four-and-a-half years since commencing university study, I graduated with two degrees from two separate universities. I then completed my Honours Degree at a hospital-based research and commercial facility. It was this experience and the mentoring and nurturing I received from a wide variety of researchers, from different professions and all at different career stages, that I was firmly decided on becoming a career health researcher. This is still an experience which I often refer to as the best year in my life (so far!); it was extremely challenging, both intellectually and professionally, but so rewarding!

Having spent a year completing my Honours qualification and as a qualified health professional, I decided that in order to develop all my skills and convert my university education into a professional set of skills, I took 12 months away from research and was employed in the health profession full time. In reflection, I am glad that I did this, as it allowed me time to consider my career direction, apply for postgraduate scholarships, and, of course, develop invaluable clinical skills.

At present, having been awarded a nationally competitive scholarship, I am now mid-way through my PhD. I'm still maintaining my clinical skills by working as often as my PhD commitments will allow me.

PhD EXPERIENCE

The PhD experience is like no other; sometimes you can be absolutely flat out and under the pump, and at other times, you can feel that you are drifting in a big ocean, looking for anything to indicate where to head towards next. I enjoy the autonomy of the PhD, especially after working full time for 12 months as a health professional! It can be an extremely isolating experience; even though you may have other researchers around you, no one else is doing exactly what you are doing and they have their own projects and research focus. I have recently had the opportunity to complete a joint project with a fellow PhD student; that continual interaction and sharing the weight of the project with someone else was such a respite from the solitude.

A PhD is a constantly moving thing; you can have a plan, but, in order to excel in this career, I think you need to be highly adaptable. Things can change so quickly; you may not get access to the particular data you need, or funding. Sometimes, there may be a difference in where you see your project heading and where your supervisor sees it going, and that interface can be quite challenging to navigate and a source of great frustration at times.

BEYOND THE PhD

I think in order to get through your PhD and out the other side (especially in a timely manner), you need to be very focussed, yet adaptable. You need to keep your eye on the horizon. Upon completion of my PhD, I hope to move overseas to complete a post-doc. It will be a great opportunity professionally and personally – that is what I am looking forward to.

Beyond completing a post-doc, I'd like to consider that I would be established as a health researcher both locally and internationally. Although I have key interests professionally which I intend to maintain, I would like to be involved in research across the health spectrum; variety is important to me. I look forward to being involved in identifying and developing the research career of other young researchers, just as my mentors have done for me.

FACTORS IN MY SUCCESS

- Not deciding too early what I wanted to do in my career, keeping a number of options open.
- Having a variety of experiences and qualifications to separate myself from my competitors.
- Being open to opportunities that present themselves, even if the timing may not be quite right.
- Not being too afraid to present my research at national conferences regularly, beginning from when I worked as a research assistant.
- Identifying mentors and being open to their advice and receptive when they share their knowledge.
- Maintaining good professional relationships with a variety of researchers.

MAJOR HURDLES

- Having confidence in myself and my own abilities.
- Finding a niche to place oneself in the big wide research world.
- Being accepted as a young researcher and forging paths into an established national research scene.

PERSONAL REFLECTION 6: LUCY BRENNAN, PhD CANDIDATE, DIVISION OF HEALTH SCIENCES, UNIVERSITY OF SOUTH AUSTRALIA, AUSTRALIA

A SURPRISE CAREER MOVE

My research journey began after a conversation I had with my Honours supervisor towards the end of my undergraduate Bachelor of Applied Science (Occupational Therapy) degree. I was asked if I had ever considered undertaking a PhD. I was surprised, as I had never considered my potential to achieve this level of postgraduate study.

During my years of undergraduate study, I had identified a career interest in academic work, knowing that a clinical career on its own may not continue to hold the challenges that I was seeking. Whilst completing my Honours research, I recognised the enjoyment I received from the challenge of conceptualising complex research problems and solutions. As I discussed with my supervisor, this element of 'challenge' that I was seeking in my work could be further facilitated through completing a higher research degree. It was this realisation that allowed me to consider embarking on a PhD.

Making the decision to apply for a PhD proved isolating in some ways. I did not receive the support I had expected from my peers. In addition, many individuals I knew who were working towards a PhD had already developed their professional identity and had not taken the same path as I was choosing. I did, however, receive invaluable support from the research team that I was hoping to join – sharing their experiences and listening to their advice about how to view this major undertaking. After meeting with my current supervisor and discussing a research topic, I developed a proposal and applied for an Australian Postgraduate Award with Stipend Scholarship, which I was successful in achieving and commenced my candidature in February 2005.

Currently, I am 18 months into my candidacy, with the aim of completing on time at the end of three years. At the beginning of this degree, my supervisor and I identified goals to develop my skills in public health theory and research to support my future research career. I commenced the appropriate course work and completed a Graduate Certificate in Public Health within my first year of candidacy.

Along with undertaking various stages of my research, I have attended two international and two national conferences. These experiences not only facilitated a comprehension of the standards and expectations of presenting at these forums, but also provided a valuable opportunity to liaise with international researchers, develop understanding of their research foci and also investigate potential opportunities for post-doctoral study.

WHAT UNDERPINS SUCCESS?

There are a number of personal and professional factors that I believe underpin success when embarking on a higher research degree and further research career:

- *Maintaining a clear view of career and life goals.* Spend time thinking about how the completion of a higher research degree will facilitate achieving what you want in the future. Remember to write these reasons down, as you will need to refer to these later down the track when extra motivation is required.
- *Keeping life in balance.* Ensure that, along with the commitment you make to a higher research degree or research career, you also make a commitment to look after your personal and social lives.
- *Maintaining a profile in discipline of training and research area of interest.* When considering applying for grants and publishing your work, be mindful of maintaining a profile in multiple professional arenas. This will facilitate greater opportunities for collaboration and potential future career advancement.
- *Mentors and supervisors.* Before commencing your research degree, ensure that you have identified appropriate mentors and supervisors. Acknowledge that the people involved in your supervision will bring different experience, skills and capacities. With this in mind, having at least two supervisors will not only increase the chances of obtaining the supervision you require, but also help you consider differing perspectives in the development of your research.
- *Standing apart from the rest.* Throughout your career, you need to consider how you can stand apart from other researchers within your discipline, institution and on a national and international scale. Identify the gaps in expertise and make the right moves to fill these. This will help to ensure the longevity of your research profile.

THE MAJOR HURDLES

There are a number of hurdles or 'challenges' that can be faced in developing a research career. These are some of the issues that I have faced since commencing my candidacy:

- *Developing a research career parallel to a clinical career.* An initial hurdle that I faced was my concern about not having time to develop a clinical career parallel to developing my research experience. I have addressed this issue by working one day a week in a clinical role, with the rest of my time focussed on my PhD commitments.
- *Confidence in own skills and abilities.* During some periods of my candidacy, I have been faced with complex issues to resolve that have not only

challenged my intellectual capacity, but, in some cases, have also caused me to question my own skills and abilities. I have since realised, however, that this career path provides challenges that you are not always meant to know the answer to. At each step along the journey, you gather valuable lessons and experiences. These, in combination with hard work, allow you to develop an excellent foundation for a future research career.

- *Maintaining motivation and focus.* With any long-term commitment, it can be difficult to maintain the same level of motivation throughout the entire process. Sometimes, you can feel lost in a pile of articles to read or numerous patients to interview. Taking time to regularly review your progress and set both short and long-term goals can help keep your eye on the horizon.

WHAT I WANT TO ACHIEVE

As a researcher, 18 months into my PhD candidacy, the most obvious goal that I have at this time is to submit my thesis and be successful in attaining a PhD. It is important, however, to keep in mind what lies ahead. At this early stage in my career, I have identified a number of career interests, including academic work and ongoing research involvement. I would like to build a reputable research and academic profile and have the opportunity to mentor others in the development of their own research careers. There are a number of paths that I could take to achieve these goals, with one approach being to apply for a post-doctoral position to further build skills and experience.

With all the career decisions that lie in front of me, it is important to acknowledge that my choices are presently guided by the potential opportunities, variety and job satisfaction that each career move may provide in the future. What I am hoping however, is that by making the early move into a research career, I will support the achievement of my personal and professional potential and a continual enjoyment of the challenges that lie ahead.

PERSONAL REFLECTION 7: ANDREA DRISCOLL, PhD CANDIDATE, SCHOOL OF NURSING, DEAKIN UNIVERSITY, MELBOURNE, AUSTRALIA

I am currently undertaking my PhD, supported by a National Health & Medical Research Council Public Health Postgraduate Research Scholarship and a National Heart Foundation of Australia grant. I am also currently a Heart Failure Nurse Practitioner candidate and run a Nurse Practitioner project at a large acute metropolitan hospital. I am at the beginning of my research career and about to complete my PhD but am at the pinnacle of my clinical career (once endorsed as a nurse practitioner).

I have been nursing for many years, specialising in cardiac nursing. In addition to working, I also undertake several professional activities outside of work hours to enhance my curriculum vitae. I am Editor of *Critical Times* (national publication of Australian College of Critical Care Nurses) and have been for over five years, and an editorial board member of *Australian Critical Care* journal. I am a consultant and expert advisor on Nurse Practitioners for the Nurses Board of Victoria. In addition to this, I also peer-review journal articles for publication for national and international journals, grade abstracts for national conferences and have been invited to judge research/scholarship nursing prizes at Australian and New Zealand Intensive Care Society national conferences and am also an invited speaker at national conferences. I have also examined and audited several Nursing Honours theses and developed a curriculum and authored several distance education subjects for a Postgraduate Certificate.

My PhD is a large national study aimed at developing national benchmarks for chronic heart failure management programmes. Fifty sites have been recruited to participate in the study and approximately 1200 patients enrolled. Currently, I am feverishly looking for employment in the field of cardiac research as a post-doctoral research fellow once I have completed my PhD. I have also applied for several post-doctoral research fellowships. The reason for applying for the fellowship is mainly the prestige of receiving a fellowship; it certainly enhances your curriculum vitae tremendously. Also, if you are successful, the fellowship pays your wage and, in research, any research institute will employ you if they don't have to pay your wage. If I am not successful in receiving a fellowship, then I will apply for an advertised research fellow position and apply the following year. You have up to five years after completing your PhD to apply for a post-doctoral fellowship. I do believe that if you want a career in research, then receiving a fellowship would put you one step ahead of your peers when applying for competitive research grants. However, having said that, the fellowships are very competitive and only a few people are awarded them annually.

One you have finished your PhD, the major objectives to achieve as quickly as possible are:

- apply for a Post-Doctoral Fellowship;
- write and publish as many articles as possible;
- apply for competitive research grants; and
- find yourself a research team to work with.

Some very wise advice that I received a couple of years ago was that 'no one is successful on their own, everyone works within a team and the team is successful'. If you look at research publications and competitive grant winners, they all work within a team, with some very high-profile and successful people in their team. I was very fortunate during my PhD in that I and fellow PhD students collaborated on writing several research papers. I sought people out in the workplace who were interested in writing papers together, as, often, you all have different ideas on a topic that would together create a good paper.

One major factor to success, I believe, is to have a mentor. In nursing, mentors are 'few and far between'; however, I know of numerous people in prestigious positions who all had mentors to advise and guide their careers. It is often through your professional network and showcasing your research that you will find a mentor. I was very fortunate with one of my supervisors for my PhD in that he gave me fantastic advice and support, and guided my PhD project into one that was of national significance.

Other factors for success are being politically astute, knowing who the major players are, avoiding getting mixed up with other people's personal agendas, and having the ability to sell yourself to anyone. Selling yourself is very difficult to do but very important, as no one else will do it for you and if you want to succeed, then people must know who you are. Publications and conference presentations are a way to raise your profile. This is all about Bob Hawke's (a former Australian Prime Minister) philosophy 'jobs for my mates'. You would be surprised what a major player networking is in making or breaking your career. Unfortunately, I am not very good at networking and selling myself at the present stage.

My career goal is to become a Professor in Nursing, to be respected for my high standard of work ethic and to have the opportunity to supervise other PhD students. However, in order to achieve this goal, I must first successfully complete my PhD and then publish, publish, publish, and network, network, network, whilst also applying for competitive research grants. Sounds busy – well, a successful career also involves plenty of hard work. Unfortunately, my PhD is not the end of my career, but only the beginning.

PERSONAL REFLECTION 8: KERENA ECKERT, PhD CANDIDATE, FACULTY OF HEALTH SCIENCES, UNIVERSITY OF QUEENSLAND, QUEENSLAND, AUSTRALIA

A SERIES OF DETOURS FROM MY CHOSEN PATH

I commenced my working career as an enrolled nurse in a private hospital and transferred shortly after gaining registration to student nurse training in the public hospital system in the belief that this would provide me with more career opportunities. After graduating as an RN, I spent several years in adult intensive and coronary care, but, due to a lack of available places in the only intensive care course in the state, I was unable to progress my education further and decided to change career directions and do my midwifery training. At the time, research did not receive much attention in nursing; nor did it feature prominently in newly developed university degree courses for nurses. Nursing embraced the idea of research and evidence-based medicine somewhat later than other disciplines, such as medicine. As one of my medical colleagues so aptly put it some years ago, 'nursing is still in the teenager phase of its research development and lags some 15 years behind us'. It is my current opinion that nursing still has a long way to go to bridge the gap.

I then spent a decade or so working as a midwife, mainly in the neonatal intensive care unit and women's emergency department of a metropolitan hospital, until, one day, I was approached and asked if I was interested in doing some part-time research for a senior obstetrician and medical director of the hospital. I jumped at the opportunity to do something different and the flexible hours were a bonus, as I had two small babies. Little did I know that this decision would be my first step on my research career path! Here, I gained my early computer (and database) research skills and, after a time, the close working relationship I had with one of the hospital specialists led to my being offered a position as a research midwife in the hospital's university department of obstetrics and gynaecology.

I remember this part of my research career as intellectually challenging but also extremely rewarding. It was also very exciting working at the cutting edge of new knowledge and it satisfied my inquisitive nature. Here, I gained valuable research skills, coordinating several drug trials and in-house randomised–controlled trials which provided me with a strong research foundation. At the suggestion of my supervisor, I enrolled in a Masters of Public Health (MPH) degree. I still remember the difficulty I experienced writing my first 5000-word essay (my nursing training certainly didn't provide me with any clues and, anyway, that was too long ago) and the pain associated with losing eight hours of edits on the computer the night before it was due to be handed up! My MPH also helped me to gain important additional skills in epidemiology and biostatistics, and overcome my major frustration of not being able to interpret or understand journal articles. It was here, under the careful nurturing and direction of one of the department professors (who later became my MPH supervisor and first career mentor), that I gained a love and passion for research which persists to this day. However, after six enjoyable years, my research career came to an abrupt end when, as part a cost-cutting exercise, the hospital decided to no longer provide support to the university for my position. I heard later that the funds were redirected to support a part-time epidemiologist! I could continue on but only in a part-time capacity, supported by a finite pool of research funds. This was not going to get my children's school fees paid for! Thus started the next phase of my career, which, on reflection, was a slight (but extremely beneficial) detour off my chosen path.

In the pursuit of permanent full-time employment, I successfully secured a position in a Department of Health as a nurse epidemiologist in the area of infectious diseases. Although I was sad leaving my research position, I was excited at the prospect of expanding the public health skills I had gained during my MPH, particularly in epidemiology and biostatistics. While infectious diseases may not be everyone's preferred career option, I would highly recommend it if you wish to gain valuable skills in applied (field) epidemiology. In my opinion, you do not appreciate the powerful contribution that epidemiology can make to the course of disease until you experience the adrenaline-pumping effects of being involved in an epidemic outbreak investigation in which decisions change, sometimes hourly, as new epidemiological evidence comes to light. Needless to say, it is a highly demanding task and, after becoming proficient in disease surveillance, managing regional databases and field epidemiology over several years, I felt it was time for a change of pace. I was also particularly frustrated at the lack of time available to write up and publish the results of my outbreak research. However, as fate would have it, another valuable opportunity surfaced and I was asked to apply for, and successfully obtained, a two-year position as an epidemiologist in the area of population health, specifically rural and remote health. Little did I know that by accepting this position, I would re-ignite my research career!

My new position was a collaborative research venture between the Department of Health and the Professor of Rural Health. I remember it well when I received an email from the professor on my very first day, suggesting that I consider using this research as a PhD. I had only just finished writing up my Masters thesis and I wasn't sure if I should 'take the plunge' again, particularly given that it had taken me over half a decade to complete the degree part time. I remember thinking 'do I want a life?' or 'do I want a PhD?'. Given my love of research, the latter position won out, of course, and I worked in this position for about a year, developing my skills in rural health epidemiology and managing large state-wide databases. After about 12 months, my PhD supervisor asked me if I was interested in applying for an academic position at the university as a research fellow. This position involved setting up an epidemiology and biostatistical consultancy for staff and students and, although particularly challenging and rewarding, it involved a very heavy workload, large amount of after-hours work and little time to spend on my PhD. So, after about a year, and with the help of my PhD supervisor, I successfully secured two scholarships to enable me to complete my PhD studies full time. I couldn't believe my luck – fancy working full time on my PhD AND being paid to do this. The scholarships enabled me to devote considerable time to my PhD and I supplemented my wage with some part-time work assisting other students with their PhDs. About 12 months into the scholarship, and nearing the final write-up stage of my thesis, I was again presented with another career opportunity that led to my current academic position. My supervisor had secured a large NHMRC grant to undertake a project but, due to unfortunate circumstances, the leading investigator could no longer be involved and, as a result, I was offered the opportunity to manage the project as part of a post-doctoral research fellowship.

MAJOR FACILITATORS AND BARRIERS TO SUCCESS

I think one of the most important things to launching a successful research career is to complete your PhD as quickly and as early in your career as possible. I remember presenting my Masters research at the university department of General Practice research colloquium, my supervisor and I being approached by several GPs in the audience who remarked that with a little more work, my Masters research would be worthy of a PhD. I declined their offer to upgrade to a PhD, thinking it more important to have an MPH, as I didn't have an undergraduate degree. I was similarly offered another opportunity a few months later to pursue a PhD on a different topic but, again, declined, but for financial reasons this time. Although I felt my reasons were valid at the time, I later regretted my decisions. Had I taken up these opportunities, I would have arrived where I am much earlier. Furthermore, while it is often necessary for financial reasons to combine PhD studies with full-time employment, I have found that this is not the best way to go. It is much harder to focus on a PhD after a long and tiring day's work and, as a PhD is a major undertaking (believe me, it is), it deserves your full attention.

I also feel that the quality of supervision is paramount to success. Shortly after I commenced my PhD, my supervisor moved inter-state. I did not feel that others at my university had adequate content knowledge and it was not possible to recruit another qualified person at another university without payment. As such, I transferred my candidature to my supervisor's university inter-state as a remote student. This was the right decision for me and has enabled me to continue my association with my supervisor, enhanced my PhD and led to important further career opportunities. Despite this, there is a downside to being a remote student – PhD isolation. While I appreciate that this is a well known phenomenon associated with PhD work, it is more acute with remote candidature. Had I not had the depth of research experience and ability to work independently, I would not have survived. However, I really miss the personal face-to-face contact and the ability to bounce things off my supervisor. So, for the majority of you who have their supervisor down the hall, do not take this for granted.

Another important issue and related to the above is one of professional isolation. Not physically being located in an academic department means that you are not surrounded by other like-minded individuals and cannot attend department seminars or establish connections and introductions with others in your field. I have found this particularly difficult but have found some solace in establishing and maintaining relationships and working on collaborative projects with several other PhD students who are in a similar position. I plan to correct this deficit by having a productive post-doc and building a track record and research profile (including attending conferences) that will position me well for future funding and research opportunities.

ACHIEVEMENTS?

When I was first asked to write this piece, my initial thought was 'I don't think I have achieved much'. On reflection, I am wrong. Indeed, this exercise has made me realise that I have come a long way from performing various procedures in the neonatal intensive care unit and questioning why this was done or whether they were beneficial. Two major achievements come immediately to mind – conquering the world of computers and statistics at a time at which most nurses had not taken the leap and completing my MPH after a long break from study and no undergraduate degree to prepare me for the transition. For those whose research careers progress in a rather orderly fashion, such as from an undergraduate degree, through an Honours programme and then PhD (perhaps with some part-time clinical experience along the way), my journey to my current academic research position may seem somewhat convoluted. It is, but much was dictated by the times, opportunity and life choices along the way. Some may think that I have pursued a research career rather too late in the piece. Others, not familiar with my background, may wonder why I have not progressed further along the university, academic research career 'highway' compared with others of my age – fancy doing a post-doc now! I can only blame a few rather interesting career detours along the way, an early career mentor who instilled in me a love of research and my current PhD supervisor's encouragement and faith in my abilities.

Research may not suit everyone. It requires passion and attention to detail. It certainly is not for the faint-hearted – coming out of a grant-writing exercise can add years to your life! Some will be in the right place at the right time, with the right mentor and career opportunities to advance rapidly through the ranks, reaching a professorial appointment in their late 30s or early 40s. For the rest of us, I suspect, our research career paths will be less grandiose. It will be harder for women with family obligations to get there. However, research can provide you with the most rewarding experience of a lifetime. If I had to do it over, I may choose a more direct path but then I wouldn't have had such an interesting journey. I am sure the next phase will be just as rewarding.

PERSONAL REFLECTION 9: MELINDA CARRINGTON, PhD CANDIDATE, PSYCHOLOGY, UNIVERSITY OF MELBOURNE, MELBOURNE, AUSTRALIA

PERSONAL BIOGRAPHY

Between 1995 and 1997, I undertook a three-year Bachelor of Arts Degree at The University of Melbourne, majoring in Criminology and Psychology. I had a one-year break from study in 1998 and then returned to The University of Melbourne in 1999 to complete a Postgraduate Diploma in Psychology. My field of research was in sleep physiology, under the supervision of Professor John Trinder. My thesis investigated the cardiovascular changes that were due to sleep and circadian (24-hour) effects. After achieving first-class honours during my fourth year of study, I commenced my PhD candidature with the same supervisor mid-way through 2000. My PhD thesis assessed cardiovascular activity during the sleep-onset period and the influence of arousals from sleep. I was awarded a Melbourne Research Scholarship in 2002 and worked on my thesis in both part-time and full-time capacities before submitting it in January 2006. My thesis is currently under examination.

WHERE I'M AT IN MY RESEARCH CAREER

I attained a post-doctoral research position with the Baker Heart Research Institute mid-way through 2005, initially on a part-time basis whilst I was in the final stages of completing my PhD. This position is responsible for assisting with the design, conduct and analysis for the Second Australian National Blood Pressure (ANBP2) Cohort Study, and it also involves managing a programme of core research from different sites in Melbourne, aimed at characterising and identifying predictors of the rate of morning surge in blood pressure in a large patient group using ambulatory blood pressure monitoring. More recently, I began working with Professor Simon Stewart on the topic of community prevention and improving health outcomes for cardiovascular disease.

The duties that I have performed in these roles have assisted my career development greatly. These responsibilities include:

- preparing grant applications to undertake new projects;
- preparing manuscripts and communications;
- managing ethics applications, amendments and progress reports;
- preparing and managing financial budgets;
- developing protocols and study databases;
- student supervision of Honours projects.

MAJOR FACTORS THAT UNDERPIN SUCCESS

I believe that young scientists are initially reliant on their supervisors for getting a good start to their career. This calls for the need to have a 'mentor' who actively encourages the inclusion of their post-doctoral fellows in activities that include preparing manuscripts and grant-funding applications, beginning in the latter stages of their PhD candidature. Grant writing is an essential skill for all scientists and should be strongly supported.

Authorship is the primary basis for assessing a scientist's contribution to developing new knowledge. Thus, communicating the results that emanate from research projects is an important aspect to becoming a successful researcher. Public presentations are another way of communicating scientific findings and it is important to be able to effectively and confidently present and defend one's results. Both these activities give rise to public exposure, promote an environment for collaboration and encourage interaction with others in the field, which, in the future, may lead to substantial scientific achievements.

MAJOR HURDLES

The major hurdles that I have encountered would relate to changing direction after my PhD and being in a workplace environment which is not oriented towards the field of research that I was trained in – that is physiological sleep research. To pursue my interest in sleep research, I believe, would have meant taking up a post-doctoral research position in the USA, which I was not interested in doing at that time. As a consequence of not integrating my sleep knowledge with my current position, I feel as though I lag behind other post-doctoral fellows who have continued to progress with their original area of research and am less 'independent' as a researcher who needs to become familiar with a new area of study.

Up until recently, when I applied for post-doctoral research fellowships and applications for research funding from granting bodies, I had only slight experience in these activities. I believe that this should have been a priority whilst in the latter stages of my PhD candidature, to assist with future success with grant and fellowship applications. To this end, having only a moderate publication record has also not been beneficial for receiving fellowship funding awards.

WHAT I HOPE TO ACHIEVE

I wish for a successful future research career and a strong ability to carry out research, both independently and as part of a team. I aspire to becoming a self-funded independent researcher and playing a prominent role in my chosen area of research. More specifically and related to my newly chosen field of research, I seek to acquire skills in order to provide the community with evidence of the effectiveness of medical interventions into the prevention of cardiovascular disease, and to carry out research that allows a better determination of the different approaches to cardiovascular disease prevention. Based on the high incidence of cardiovascular disease in Australia, I want to create a healthier environment for Australians and educate the general public about cardiovascular health and well-being.

PERSONAL REFLECTION 10: GERALDINE LEE, PhD CANDIDATE, UNIVERSITY COLLEGE LONDON, UNITED KINGDOM

I commenced hospital-based nurse training in London in 1987. Throughout my training, I worked on medical, surgical, obstetric and psychiatric wards;

however, the area that interested me the most was coronary care. Being based in central London at St Bartholomew's Hospital, patients were transferred with heart failure, unstable arrhythmias and those awaiting surgery. One of the issues that interested me was the different responses of patients to cardiac medications. Consequently, I enrolled in a Bachelor of Science Physiology degree at University College London, which incorporated physiology, pathophysiology and pharmacology. Students from several disciplines undertook lectures: medicine, anatomy, pharmacology and biomedical sciences. With my special interest in cardiology, I chose a laboratory-based project for my Honours and examined global ischaemia in the isolated rat heart. The benefits of studying at UCL was the high standard of academics, the clinical focus of the course with practising consultants presenting sessions and the opportunity to undertake PhDs, etc. with world experts (one of my lecturers was Professor Steve Jones, known for his books and television documentaries on genetics).

The benefits of undertaking a physiology degree and laboratory work were several and I have a much better understanding of the clinical application of physiology and pathophysiology. This integration of theory to practice really benefited my patient care and I was able to organise teaching sessions for nursing staff and patients.

Although I enjoyed working as a nurse in coronary care, my interest in research was not satisfied and I consequently undertook a nursing research position investigating a neuro-protective agent in patients undergoing coronary artery bypass graft surgery (CABGS). The study was a randomised–controlled trial in association with a pharmaceutical company and University College London was paired with Duke University in the USA. The research project involved recruiting patients from the pre-admission clinic, carrying out a thorough assessment prior to their operation and following them up postoperatively. All patients underwent neuropsychological assessment to determine their concentration, memory and attention. During the operation, transcranial Doppler monitoring was performed which demonstrated the presence of micro-emboli (associated with neuropsychological decline in CABGS patients). From this project, I began my PhD, examining patient-perceived quality of life five years after CABGS, based at the Centre for Behavioural Sciences at UCL and working with health psychologists. The aspects that I studied involved use of quality-of-life questionnaires, diet and physical activity questionnaires and psychological well-being examining depression and anxiety. Patients and their respective spouses were invited to participate in this follow-up study and a total of 118 patients participated. Combining the patients' and spouses' perspectives (subjective data) with clinical objective data (such as angina and breathlessness) demonstrated the advantages of collecting both types of data.

Of course, no research is complete without statistical analysis. This, I have to admit, was the most difficult part of my thesis. I set up my database and basically taught myself statistical skills (no mean feat!). Although I wouldn't call myself a statistical 'expert', I am confident about interpreting statistics and know my limitations. It is important to remember that there are statistical experts available in most universities and the internet is an excellent source of information.

Doctoral studies can be quite frustrating, with highs and lows. As nurses, we are very task-oriented and changing to an analytical and 'cerebral' approach was much harder than I imagined. My fellow psychology doctoral students were quite comfortable doing a literature search and reading two or three articles in a day. I had to accept that this, in academic terms, is a good day! I was fortunate that the department had a dozen PhD students so peer support was always available as well as monthly journal clubs in which we presented our research and discussed issues. I have enjoyed undertaking my thesis and have seen it as a huge learning curve. It isn't easy, but perseverance is certainly required.

In 2001, I moved to Melbourne, Australia, and commenced lecturing at La Trobe University. Luckily, I have been based at the Alfred Hospital, where clinical research opportunities abound. I have been able to investigate clinical issues in cardiac, cardiothoracic and emergency nursing, presenting findings at national and international conferences and supervising Honours and Masters nursing students.

I have now completed my PhD and am awaiting an oral viva to defend my thesis (standard practice for UK doctoral studies). One of the amazing things that happened was meeting with Professor Stewart at the Cardiac Society of Australia and New Zealand conference earlier this year. Consequently, I am about to start post-doctoral studies at the Baker Heart Research Institute in Melbourne in cardiovascular studies. Having examined so many variables that can affect individuals, I can now appreciate the importance of pathophysiology, psychological well-being, social support and dietary behaviour in those with cardiovascular conditions.

My aim since I started nursing was to improve patient outcomes, improve quality of life and educate patients and their families about coronary heart disease. One way of doing this is through working on a ward, doing clinical shifts, and another way is through research. I hope that through the research pathway, a greater impact can occur. It is an interesting journey, with many challenges on the way. I have to admit that when I undertook the physiology degree, it was purely for selfish reasons, as I wanted to improve my understanding in this field. My other passion is writing and this is certainly beneficial when it comes to writing research papers.

To succeed, a novice researcher needs peer support, a role model, regular contact with supervisors and a forum to discuss research issues and problems. Research should be a collaborative, multidisciplinary, enjoyable experience and working in a team can be very rewarding. Health research allows health professionals to amalgamate theory to practice and hopefully make a difference. I would suggest to anyone interested in research to get actively involved, as there are always opportunities to gain experience.

PERSONAL REFLECTION 11: Dr CRAIG HANSEN, BSc (PUBLIC HEALTH) (HONS), PhD (ENVIRONMENTAL EPIDEMIOLOGY)

A POST-DOCTORAL POINT OF VIEW

My first career was teaching music in private schools and, after being in the industry for almost a decade, I had a strong desire to change careers. I was always interested in establishing a career in health; however, the broad spectrum of different opportunities available within the health sector generated uncertainty regarding the area of health that I wanted to pursue. After investigating various possible pathways, I decided to study public health, and, in retrospect, this was driven by my desire to be involved in health at a population level as opposed to an individual level. My undergraduate degree involved studying a diverse range of subjects, including life sciences, environmental health, health promotion and epidemiology/biostatistics. It was the latter, however, that gained my strongest interest and respect, as I enjoyed analysing health data. To me, epidemiology and biostatistics is the 'nuts and bolts' or the 'backbone' of health research, as the challenge is to *make sense* of the data by correctly collecting, preparing, analysing, interpreting and reporting what the data are trying to tell us.

My other area of interest was environmental health, so I decided to marry the two areas of interest together and carry out my doctorate in environmental epidemiology, in which I investigated the effect of ambient air pollution during pregnancy on birth outcomes. This was, and still is, a reasonably new area of research, which made it quite challenging, yet very rewarding. Due to this area of research's being in its infancy, and to my advantage, there was a wide variety of government and non-government sectors that displayed great interest in my research.

I am currently at the post-doctoral stage of my research career, in which I am involved in several projects that encompass very different areas of health. The projects I am currently involved in are: (1) cardiovascular disease among the black population of Soweto, South Africa – the primary aim of this research 'is to systematically examine the epidemiologic transition in risk behaviours and clinical presentations of heart disease in the predominantly Black African population of approximately one million people living in the townships that comprise the internationally renowned and celebrated area of Soweto' (Stewart *et al.*, 2006); (2) investigating surgical margins in the treatment of non-melanoma skin cancer in Australia – the primary aim of this research is to assess skin cancer pathology reports and analyse the margins of excision along with the number of pigmented skin lesions excised per melanoma (referred to as the 'number needed to treat'); and (3) assessing the impact of ambient air pollution on birth defects and fetal ultrasonic measures among pregnancies – this research is a continuation of the research conducted for my doctorate and is very important, as no previous studies have been able to establish how fetal growth patterns may vary in relation to ambient air pollution during pregnancy.

Although my research career is only young, the diverse range of projects that I am currently involved in will allow me to expand and grow in many different facets of health research. These include establishing and maintaining professional partnerships at national and international levels, managing and analysing different types of health data, authoring quality scientific publications to different audiences, and gaining recognition within various areas of research. I consider all of these facets as key aspects of success and, most importantly, a productive post-doctoral stage provides the recognition and expertise to become an independent researcher, which is one of the standout aspects to becoming a successful researcher.

As with any career path, there are often many hurdles that need jumping (or passing under – lateral thinking!); however, I can only go by experience and, therefore, I would like to point out several hurdles in the very early stage of a research career. Although this may seem obvious, but the very first hurdle is to successfully complete a doctorate whereby the topic is of interest to yourself and a particular audience and, in addition, there needs to be the potential for further research within your topic, or the potential to expand to other areas. I consider this to be a vital stage in establishing a career in health research, as it is the period during which the seed is planted for your research career to potentially sprout and grow (with a little nurturing). Another hurdle is the personal adjustment from being a doctoral candidate to a post-doctorate. As in my case, and I assume in many others, the post-doctoral projects are in different areas of health from my doctorate study and, while this is a great way to expand your career prospects, it can also be overwhelming, as you need to establish new contacts and networks, familiarise yourself with the latest literature and study methods, and gain the respect of a new group of researchers. The biggest and most challenging hurdle when starting a research career is to obtain financial funding through various research grants. It is often required that young researchers first apply for small grants or be part of a research team comprising more established researchers who have prior experience and success with research grants.

Finally, as with any career, there is always the 'big' question of 'what do you hope to achieve in your career?'. It is intuitively appealing to state that you hope to achieve substantial recognition within your field whereby it provides you with the opportunity of continuous funding for ongoing research projects as well as a prosperous career. However, with some further thought, this question is not always easy to answer.

Despite its importance in establishing a successful and satisfying research career, I feel that climbing the academic ladder and gaining professional notoriety through a wealth of publications and conference presentations should not always be viewed as the only way to success. I feel that success is also achieving the personal fulfilment of improving people's health and quality of life, which is the main rationale for health research.

REFERENCE

Stewart S, Wilkinson D, Becker A, Askew D, Ntyintyane L, McMurray JJ and Sliwa K. (2006) Mapping the emergence of heart disease in a black, urban population in Africa: The Heart of Soweto Study. *International Journal of Cardiology* 108: 101–108.

PERSONAL REFLECTION 12: Dr DIEM DINH, POST-DOCTORAL FELLOW, BAKER HEART RESEARCH INSTITUTE, MELBOURNE, AUSTRALIA

My interest in a scientific research career began in my teens, when my dad was diagnosed with high blood pressure and his father died of a stroke. I started my undergraduate degree in medical lab science and subsequently obtained an Honours Degree in Pharmacology at RMIT University. I was then awarded a NH&MRC/Dora Lush Research Scholarship to undertake a PhD in pharmacology and molecular biology. As a recipient of the NH&MRC/CJ Martin Fellowship, I carried out my post-doctoral training overseas at the College de France (Paris) – a prestigious organisation for cardiovascular research. Upon returning to Australia, I completed my post-doc in the Molecular Endocrinology Lab at the Baker Heart Research Institute (BHRI) – the premier centre for research and training in cardiovascular diseases.

During my last year of post-doc, I re-assessed my career and decided that I wanted to learn clinical research to complement my laboratory experiences. Seizing a fortunate opportunity, I started as a project manager at the Cardiovascular Disease Prevention Unit at the Baker Heart Research Institute in Melbourne, Australia. As the name suggests, our team undertakes research that is directly relevant to improving heart disease-related health outcomes in population-based studies. I was happy with the new challenges but, at the same time, uncertain that I might not meet the high expectations or be cut out for this job. With no previous clinical research experience, it proved a steep learning curve, like being thrown into the deep. It became my responsibility to coordinate multiple projects, including clinical trials and registries. One of the main activities that I manage is the Australian Society of Cardiac and Thoracic Surgeons (ASCTS) Database Project. This programme aims to ensure that high-quality cardiac surgery is being carried out in Victorian Public Hospitals, and that the results of this surgery are being recorded and published. The transition from basic scientist to health researcher requires adaptation. I feel that my career experiences and mentors have aided in this transition process. After almost two years, I still enjoy going to work.

Attributes that determine my success in health research include perseverance, hard work and a passion for improving population health. Another key factor is having a supportive mentor, as good mentorship is critical in career development. My recommendation to younger scientists, who want to make a career in medical research, is to make the right choices from the start, including institution, hot research topics, good and successful mentors, and ensuring you put in the hard yards.

During my time as a graduate student, I observed major hurdles of securing government grants and the expectations that one must be multitalented to succeed (excel in lab management, grant writing, public speaking, teaching and research). I witnessed my very promising, talented and dedicated supervisor's short-term research career end prematurely, because he was not successful in securing further funds. The majority of my fellow colleagues left the field of research upon graduation, as they no longer had the patience or enthusiasm for the intricacy of our profession. Another key obstacle that I have experienced, especially during my PhD years, was the almost absence of social activities, but I have now learned to balance my career and non-career activities (family and friends). Although being a scientist does not offer as good a salary as some other jobs, I find my profession very satisfying and intellectually challenging. Still, medical research does offer its own rewards, like frequent travels to national and international medical conferences.

My priority now is to expand the Victorian ASCTS database project into a national database programme and eventually grow beyond the Australian waters to include New Zealand and the Asia Pacific Regions.

PERSONAL REFLECTION 13: MARY BOYDE, CLINICAL LECTURER, SCHOOL OF NURSING, THE UNIVERSITY OF QUEENSLAND, PRINCESS ALEXANDRA HOSPITAL, BRISBANE, AUSTRALIA

I am currently employed as a Clinical Lecturer/Nurse Educator with the University of Queensland and Princess Alexandra Hospital in Brisbane. I began my nursing career over 25 years ago, completing my training as a Registered Nurse in Christchurch, New Zealand. I have worked in New Zealand, New South Wales and Queensland, gaining clinical nursing experience in many fields of critical care nursing whilst specialising in coronary care nursing. I became involved in nursing education when I moved to Brisbane. Initially, I worked in staff development within a hospital setting and, over the last three years, I have worked in the School of Nursing at the University of Queensland. This is a fairly unique position, in which I teach undergraduate students for the semester and then return to work with registered nurses in a tertiary referral hospital between semesters. It is both challenging and rewarding, working across two different educational settings within the nursing profession.

Education and research are essential components of nursing. Working within education has enabled me to participate in a number of small clinically focussed research projects. I conducted a study of nurses' ability to perform cardiopulmonary resuscitation in which I completed my Masters thesis. More recently, I have investigated clinical outcomes for in-hospital cardiac arrests following the implementation of semi-automatic defibrillators in our hospital. Currently, I am researching education for heart failure patients; this is my PhD project that I started earlier this year.

Nurses at all levels need to be more involved in nursing research. I believe nursing research can create positive changes in patient care. The success of any research project is multifactorial; however, for me, one of the key underpinnings is collaboration. Research in a clinical environment needs a team of committed people who assist with the project whether it is small or large. Even from the early beginnings of a project, you need to be able to discuss the project with other interested nurses to develop a proposal. Working together as a team is necessary to sustain the project through to conclusion and then implement the findings to improve patient care. Researchers who feel supported and encouraged to continue with the project will often be successful. Working in collaboration enhances nursing research and enables us to investigate nursing practice and improve patient outcomes. Another key element is support from other nurse researchers who are more experienced and can act as mentors for the project. With each project that I have undertaken, I have been able to work with experienced nurse researchers who have initially offered guidance and then critiqued my work as I have progressed through the study. I think the role of mentors, or supervisors, as we often call them, in research is undervalued. A mentor can provide the novice nurse researcher with leadership and direction thus promoting the development of essential research skills. Within the clinical environment, it is essential that nurses who are working as clinicians establish links with experienced researchers to assist them with their research.

One of the major hurdles for nursing research is time constraints. It is a constant challenge just being able to find the time to undertake nursing research within our practice. I think nursing research needs to have a stronger focus and should be incorporated into every nursing position, with more support at an institutional level. Increased resources to support nursing research in the clinical environment would assist with the integration of research into clinical practice. I have found that inadequate time and lack of organisational support hindered my ability to undertake nursing research. My current position, which offers me the opportunity to work for a university as well as a hospital, has enhanced my ability to undertake further research. However, it is not common practice for nurses to be able to work across two settings, so we need to develop strategies to assist nurses within clinical practice settings undertake research. My aim would be to incorporate nursing research into the clinical environment and work more closely with clinicians to complete research projects, which will positively impact on patient care. A more integrated and collaborative model involving clinicians, educators and researchers would benefit the nursing practice.

SUMMARY

Clearly, this is not an exhaustive list of questions, but merely designed to provoke some final thoughts and reflection. Nor should it be considered as a 'one size fits all'. In essence, it articulates the kind of critically informed questions that will enable you to continually improve your research skills and knowledge. At every stage of your research career, you should compile your own list of questions and strategic goals in order to create your own destiny for success. As your career progresses, be prepared to re-evaluate your goals and re-engineer them to suit your circumstances (e.g. starting a family) and potential opportunities (e.g. moving overseas). The series of personal reflections provided above also provide important food for thought, as they reflect the mindset, hopes and aspirations of a number of emerging health researchers as they strive to make their mark on the academic, professional and, indeed, wider world. Hopefully, their and the above words will help guide your own journey in this regard.

Key Points: The *only* person capable of ensuring that you succeed in your chosen career path is you. To do this, it is essential you have a vision and then create the environment (a combination of supporters/mentors and strategy) to make it happen! Remember . . . 'who dares wins!'

References

Dever M, Morrison Z, Dalton B and Tayton S (2006) When research works for women. Monash University, Melbourne, ISBN 0-9756822-1-0, p ii.

Hoddell S (2000) The Professional Doctorate and the PhD: Converging or diverging lines. Presentation at the Annual SRHE conference, Sheffield, 21 December 2000.

Kirkman S, Thompson DR, Watson R and Stewart S. Are all Doctorates equal or are some 'more equal than others'? An examination of which ones should be offered by Schools of Nursing and Midwifery. *Nurse Education Today*, accepted July 2006.

Powell S (2004) The award of PhD by published work in the UK. UK Council for Graduate Education, London.

QAA (2000) The framework for higher education qualifications in England, Wales and Northern Ireland. November 2000. Quality Assurance Agency for Higher Education, Gloucester, www.qaa.uk/crntwork/nqf/ewni/contents.htm.

Simpson R (1983) How the PhD came to Britain: A century of struggle for postgraduate education. Society for Research into Higher Education, Guildford.

Stewart S, Wilkinson D, Becker A, Askew D, Ntyintyane L, McMurray JJ and Sliwa K (2006) Mapping the emergence of heart disease in a black, urban population in Africa: The Heart of Soweto Study. *International Journal of Cardiology*, 108: 101–108.

Thompson DR, Kirkman S, Watson R and Stewart S (2005) Improving research supervision in nursing. *Nurse Education Today* 25: 283–290.

Index